WHEN PIGS FLY

An Exceptional Journey

Gretchen Cooke
Jennifer Elisabeth Cooke Rinehart

History Sleuth

PHOTOGRAPHY:

Black Labs Ltd.

COVER ART:

Jessica A. Coker-Cooke

Sara M. Coker

CONSULTANT:

Aaron Cooke, Author

EDITING:

Adrian Cooke

Jessica A. Coker-Cooke

ISBN 978 0 9829999 0 5

Printed in the United States. For information address the authors @ Box 461, Arnold, MD. 21012

www.whenpigsflybook.com

e-mail: WHENPIGSFLY@historical-sleuth.com

For Tony and all fathers who are always there for their children

and

For all those who mark the box agreeing to be organ donors: your decision is a gift of life

In Memory of "Marta"
Martha Elisabeth Riis Moore
1914 - 2008

INTRODUCTION

WHEN PGS FLY is the story of an amazing young woman and her exceptional journey. A journey not taken by choice but out of necessity. Born with a rare liver defect and a life expectancy of eighteen months, she has made the journey with aplomb, grace, laughter, and love.

Historical references refer to attempts at transplantation of limbs and organs centuries earlier, but it was not until the twentieth century successful human organ transplantation became a reality. The first successful kidney transplant was performed in 1954[i], but liver transplantation was still in its infancy and not a realistic option at the time of her birth. Many years passed before liver transplantation was a viable and successful option. Paramount to this success was the vision, hard work, and scientific inquiry of physicians and medical personnel. However, the success of the procedure is meaningless without the gift of life – the donation of organs for transplantation. It is the donors and their families who have given the "gift of life" to so many in need.

The story is more than the journey of one exceptional young woman. More broadly it serves as an example of the importance of human organ donation and the unselfish gift of life donors provide to those in need.

PROLOGUE

I am young, alone, and driving one of the few cars going East on Broad Street. A stretch of Broad Street considered the "wrong side of the street" even in daylight. I am in a hurry with only one thought: to get to Jennifer.

Clouds cover the sky, and the only light is from neon signs on the storefront businesses and dim street lights. Barely enough light to separate the woman from the lamp post. Absorbed by my anxiety and fear, I am half way down the next block before I acknowledge what I had seen.

A woman, in the dark of the night, stepping away from the lamp post to the side of the curb – bending over. She did not notice it was a young woman driving – only the size and shape of the old Mercedes. The darkness shadowed the age and condition of the car – the grace and lines of the 220S signaled a potential customer.

I think occasionally, no, often, of this unknown woman. What were her circumstances? Did she survive or was she a casualty of the streets? I laugh at my naiveté and surprise. I realize in some ways she is symbolic of the road Jennifer and I would travel over the years. Faced with situations we could never have imagined, we were forced to accept and adapt to realities and situations we had never envisioned.

Much has changed in thirty-eight years. There have been incredible technological advances in science and medicine. Information, news, and communication is available twenty-four hours a day. The role of the daily newspaper is challenged: who needs the paper when they have the Internet? Much has changed, but much remains the same.

In 1972 the Eagles released their first album, Richard Nixon was President, and the United States was involved in the Vietnam War. Nixon is no longer president, but the Eagles are still playing, we are enmeshed in another war, there are still ladies of the night, and the excitement of the birth of a baby remains the same.

CHAPTER ONE

THE BEGINNING

"Jen, she has red hair. You've got your *red-headed* little girl!" Groggy from the anesthesia, she must be dreaming. Red hair? Her baby? The baby she had dreamed about, a baby with beautiful red hair like Aaron's?

It wasn't until she awoke again in recovery she realized she wasn't dreaming. The emergency C-section was over, and Chris introduced Jennifer to Isabella, their four-pound-fourteen ounce miracle. Born October 2, 2006, she arrived exactly one month early, but she was here, she was beautiful, and both Jennifer and Isabella were healthy. Ten fingers, ten toes, a head of red hair, and a lusty cry to let everyone know she had arrived.

Thirty-four years ago neither her doctors nor we had envisioned this day. How can you think of the future when you have been told there is no future? When there are many days when you are only asking for another day, another month, hoping there will be a miracle to save your baby.

Many people ask why Jennifer's story has not been told. It was a question I could never answer except to say I was too close to the situation. Jennifer is too big a part of my heart. Why now? What is different? With the birth of Isabella, Jennifer and Chris' beautiful little redheaded daughter, it is now time to share her story – a story of hope, determination, laughter, and tears. A story validating the cost and risk of organ donation for those involved in policy debates concerning health expenditures. A story to encourage people to mark the spot on their driver's license to become potential organ donors.

Jennifer and I would write jointly about the gift Jennifer received – a liver donated to Jennifer when she was eighteen. Jennifer is thirty-eight, and the ensuing years post transplant have been filled with wonderful events, as well as the usual ups and downs of life. But to an organ recipient even these ups and downs of life are wonderful – they would not have been possible without the transplant. And beautiful little Isabella would not have been possible without the liver transplant. A mother herself, Jennifer understands now how difficult it was for her parents to watch her suffer through so many surgeries and procedures.

Jennifer was beautiful – blond, petite, with long, slender fingers and toes. My first impression was pure joy. Two and a half years younger than her brother Aaron, she came into the world with a bang. A week early, labor had advanced rapidly. Every light going East on Broad to the hospital was red, and there were no police in sight. It was 1972 and cell phones were unknown to the general public. Jennifer was our second child, and we knew birth was imminent. Cautiously running the red lights, luck was with us in the form of the Hospital Administrator walking through the lobby as we arrived at the hospital. Recognizing the urgency of the situation, he commandeered the nearest elevator. She was determined and would not wait to arrive in the delivery room, making her entrance as the elevator door opened at the labor and delivery floor. I have marveled at her determination and laughed at her entrance into the world. If I were more prescient I would have realized how important Jennifer's determination and love of life would be to her survival.

She was perfect. Big blue eyes and a beautiful olive tone to her skin (the dark Danish heritage from my side of the family). Born late in the evening, we spent the hours until midnight calling friends and family. Little did we know that would be our last night of rest for many nights to come.

Our pediatrician was considered one of the top physicians in Richmond, but his bedside manner was non-existent. Barely awake I looked at my watch. It was 7:15 a.m., and Tony was at home taking care of Aaron. Standing in the doorway in his starched white coat it never occurred to him to wait until my husband was with me. Jennifer's coloring was not due to our dark Danish heritage but elevated bilirubin, or jaundice. His professional opinion? She was a very sick little baby. It was not a question of blood incompatibility. I was 0- and her father was 0+, but I had been given the RhoGam® shot to prevent complications following the birth of Aaron. His opinion was there was a major issue with the liver.

How could our beautiful little baby be ill? She threw up a few times following her birth but other than the jaundice there were no other symptoms. We were naive and innocent. We were told to take her home: it was probably neonatal jaundice. Later we realized it had been a false hope – her pediatrician had not been the only one who had suspected a major problem before she left the hospital. She would be diagnosed with biliary atresia - a very rare congenital birth defect, and her life expectancy was eighteen months. And those eighteen months? We would be lucky if she did not spend most of her short life in the hospital.

After her diagnosis of biliary atresia, a friend who was a pathologist told us he had suspected biliary atresia immediately. Unlike today, doctors were not trained to be honest with patients. Patronizing is the word that most readily comes to mind in their treatment of patients and their families. Their authority was supreme – the patient or guardian was not entitled to participate in decisions concerning treatment. They were not expected to be able to understand the medical lexicon and terminology much less the treatment options. Although there has been improvement over the years in recognition of patient's rights and ability to understand their treatment, some in the medical field still have difficulty with it. But thirty-eight years ago it was a daily battle to actively participate in Jennifer's health care.

We took Jennifer home from the hospital, but only for two short weeks. What were they like? She cried, continually. She never slept, and I never slept. Aaron spent many hours with family and friends, and her father had to resume traveling for his job. Dr. Spock,

Jennifer and I walked the floors, trying everything I read on calming a "colicky baby." I called relatives and friends for suggestions. We tried every suggestion that sounded remotely realistic as well as a few remedies that were surely old wives' tales. After not gaining weight for those two weeks, she was admitted to St. Mary's Hospital. The doctors had suspected a major problem all along and a liver biopsy confirmed the diagnosis of biliary atresia. Two weeks later she was transferred to the Medical College of Virginia Hospital (MCV), the teaching hospital where she was born, and admitted to the sick baby nursery (today these nurseries are called Neonatal Intensive Care Units (NICU). She would not return home until she was almost a year old.

What is biliary atresia? How did Jennifer end up with this devastating problem? Biliary atresia occurs when the common bile duct, leading from the liver to the gall bladder, is blocked. In addition, the bile ducts within the liver may be blocked. Bile, produced by the liver, is necessary for the digestion of food and absorption of nutrients. The normal route is from the liver to the gall bladder and then to the intestines. With blocked bile ducts, the bile is not able to leave the liver. Bile, necessary for digestion, destroys the cells of the liver if it remains in the liver. The bile backs up, causing scarring (cirrhosis) of the liver, and eventual destruction of the liver. How did Jennifer end up with biliary atresia? Even today, thirty-eight years later, there is no clear answer. Immediately after her diagnosis I was questioned about my intake of raw seafood, trips abroad, and anything unusual that may have occurred during my pregnancy. It was thought I may have acquired a mild case of hepatitis at the end of my pregnancy, and this viral illness had attacked the bile ducts of the fetus. There was no easy answer. I had not eaten raw seafood and I had not traveled abroad. Was the cold I experienced at the end of the pregnancy instead a mild case of hepatitis?

Statistically biliary atresia is more common in girls and in those of Asian and African American heritage. Approximately one in 15,000 to 20,000 babies do not have complete bile ducts. Biliary atresia can occur in uteri (before birth) or after birth[ii]. In Jennifer's case they felt it had occurred in uteri, probably during the last part of my pregnancy when the liver was formed. Jennifer had fully developed bile ducts but they were occluded. I am neither Asian nor African American. They are no closer today determining the cause of Jennifer's biliary atresia than they were thirty-eight years ago.

How to describe what the year at MCV was like? Terrifying and sterile. I was born at MCV, and from what I could see it had not changed since my birth. Located in the older section of Richmond, the main hospital where the nursery was located was one of the tallest buildings in the city. Erected in 1940, the building was a 600 bed addition to MCV, which had been established in 1838[iii]. As late as the 1970s you could walk underground via tunnels from the hospital to the State Capital and many of the other structures in downtown Richmond. As you walked huge pipes overhead creaked as they expanded and contracted. Droplets of water fell from uneven joints of the underground central steam system. Doctors and nurses, dressed formally in starched whites, moved back and forth through the tunnels to various buildings in the hospital complex. Patients, some still in the old high-backed wooden wheelchairs, rode elevators to the tunnels and were transported to different departments for treatments. Men and women in suits walked the tunnels to the different state and city buildings above ground.

The exterior of the hospital is a dark brick, designed to fit into the overall pattern of an old Southern city and matched many of the other buildings nearby. Inside, the walls were white and the floors were shining bright, but the small windows allowed little light into the building. It was sterile and not visitor friendly. Visitor lounges were few and small with unappealing furniture, and there was no lounge at all for the sick baby nursery. The main lounge was the lounge on the first floor for all those who were waiting to be admitted to the hospital.

Why would there be a lounge when visitation in the special nursery was severely restricted? Parents were not encouraged to visit except within a very limited time frame and they were never allowed to spend the night. Grandparents, siblings, and other relatives were never allowed in the nursery. We were shocked grandparents were not allowed to visit children who were often critically ill. My mother, working in an office near the hospital, would have loved to spend time but was never allowed to visit. Deciding to take Aaron away for the weekend, I begged the nurses to allow my twin sister and mother to spend time with Jennifer, but to no avail. Only parents were allowed, and only for a few hours each day. Did we go away for the weekend? No, as I could not bear the thought there would be no one to sit and hold Jennifer. The nurses were wonderful but they were unable or unwilling to bend the rules. Aaron became a regular at my twin's home, and I would spend my days at the hospital, anxiously waiting for the small increments of time I was allowed to be with Jennifer. Whenever a crisis occurred I would sleep in the waiting room of the hospital, not allowed to interrupt the routine of the nursery at night. There were a few small lounges on floors other than the first floor, and I would sneak into those lounges after visiting hours. Staying overnight anywhere in the hospital was frowned upon, but I became a familiar face to many of the night nurses. Occasionally one would quietly provide a blanket and pillow to soften the hard chairs and couches of the lobby. Ronald McDonald House would not set up housekeeping until a number of years later, and the only hotels nearby were hotels from the same era as the hospital. The once elegant Hotel Jefferson, built in the late 1890s, and the John Marshall Hotel, built in the early 1900s, were the only nearby hotels.

What was the nursery like? Sterile, with lights on twenty-four hours a day. There was the constant hum of machines pumping fluids into the sick babies, monitors checking their vital signs, and nurses moving in between the cribs. This is probably why even today, thirty-eight years later, Jennifer cannot stand to sleep with any noise or lights on. The room has to be completely dark with a fan to provide white noise. There were no chairs beside the cribs – long visits were not allowed. Two rocking chairs sat near the nurses' station – not so much for the mothers' benefit but for the nurses when they were feeding the babies. What were Jennifer's medical options as a child born in 1972 with biliary atresia? There were none. We were told we could opt for a liver transplant but they were still very experimental. The first successful human kidney transplant had been performed in 1954, but liver transplants had not achieved the same success. Still experimental, she would be lucky to survive the surgery, and if she did she would likely not live more than six months post surgery. And the six months would be in the hospital, fighting rejection of the liver. After reading what limited material was available on pediatric liver transplantation, we decided we would rather Jennifer spend what time she had with us and with her brother. If her time was going to be limited, we did not want it spent in the hospital. We asked them to do everything possible they could to make her more comfortable, short of a transplant.

With that in mind, the pediatric surgeon at the hospital made the decision to attempt some innovative surgeries. Surgeries that would not cure the biliary atresia, but would perhaps give Jennifer the chance to go home and to be with her family. Literally scraping the liver, Dr. H. M. Lee created an artificial stoma from the liver. The intention was to allow the bile to flow from the liver. Lacking healthy bile ducts, the bile was backing up in the liver. The stoma would be kept open with a piece of rubber tubing. The bile would exit the body via the stoma. No bile would be directed into the intestines but would collect in a bag over the stoma. She would still not be digesting food properly or getting the nutrients she needed. This would be addressed with a special formula and other dietary plans, but they hoped the rapid destruction of the liver by the trapped bile would be slowed.

Weighing less than six pounds and only six weeks old, Jennifer was wheeled to the operating room. Following the surgery, she was taken to the nursery from the recovery room. We were unable to hold or touch Jennifer – only to look through the plastic of the isolette where she lay, tubes connecting her to machines monitoring the functions of her body. Looking back I feel sure the nurses must have had more empathy than they exhibited, but I sometimes wonder. I have fond memories of one nurse, an LPN, who at least tried to spend time letting me know exactly what was being done and how Jennifer was responding. It was very difficult to not be able to hold and touch my beautiful daughter.

Jennifer's recovery following the surgery was a bell weather of the future. She rebounded quickly, and we looked forward to taking her home from the hospital.

We were wrong - almost ten months would elapse before we were to leave the hospital, and it was not as we had hoped. Jennifer recovered well from the surgery but developed an infection that commonly affects those with similar surgeries – ascending cholangitis. When we finally left the hospital Jennifer was eleven months old and had been running an intermittent fever up to 104 degrees for over eight months. We had decided, and her doctors concurred, they had done everything possible. It was time for Jennifer to go home to be with her family.

We were going home, and some of the children in the nursery would not go home. We met only one other child during the year with biliary atresia. The first born of a young African American couple, he did not survive past three months. The fear was always with you, and each day when I entered the nursery I would surreptitiously look around at the other cribs to see if all of Jennifer's roommates were still there. We usually knew in advance if someone was going home as there was so much excitement, and if there was an empty crib it was an ominous sign.

My Biafra baby. Are you old enough to remember the pictures, splashed over the pages of the newspapers and television, of the starving children of Biafra? Extremely thin, big eyes in gaunt faces, and big bellies. This was Jennifer, my Biafra baby. She was malnourished from the lack of nutrients and she was jaundiced, but to me she was beautiful. Years later, looking back at the picture taken the day she came home I realized how she must have appeared to those who did not know her, but to me she was perfect.

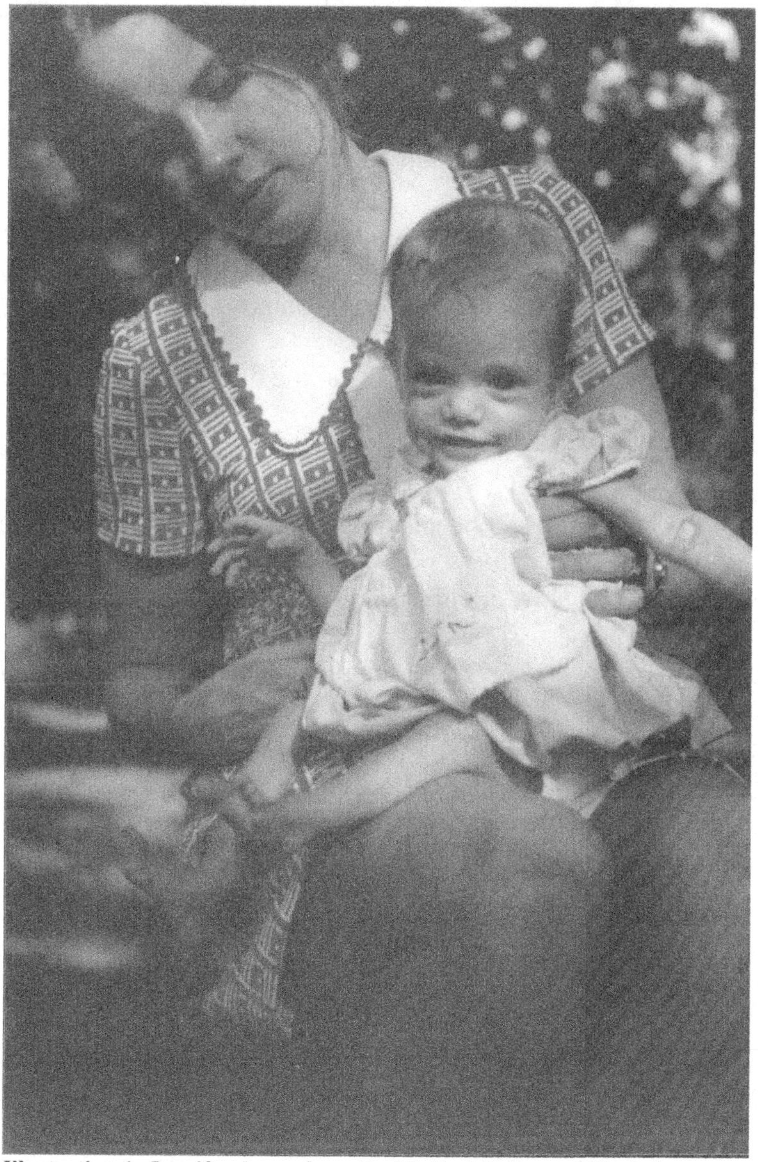

Illustration 1: Jennifer, home from the Medical College of Virginia (MCV), 1972

Was it being at home, with her family, receiving the love and attention it was impossible for her to receive in such a sterile hospital setting? Did the antibiotics finally start controlling the infection? I don't know, but I believe it was being at home with her family. She surprised everyone, especially the physicians who had sent her home. Jennifer thrived. I learned how to clean the drain, even learning how to gently replace the rubber tubing when it had slipped out of place. Leaving the hospital I had been sure I could never manage to do it – this was my baby. How could anyone expect me to put a rubber tube into the side of her body? The infection abated, or at least was under control, and the special formula (Portagen) enabled her to get some of the nutrients she needed. She grew and put on weight.

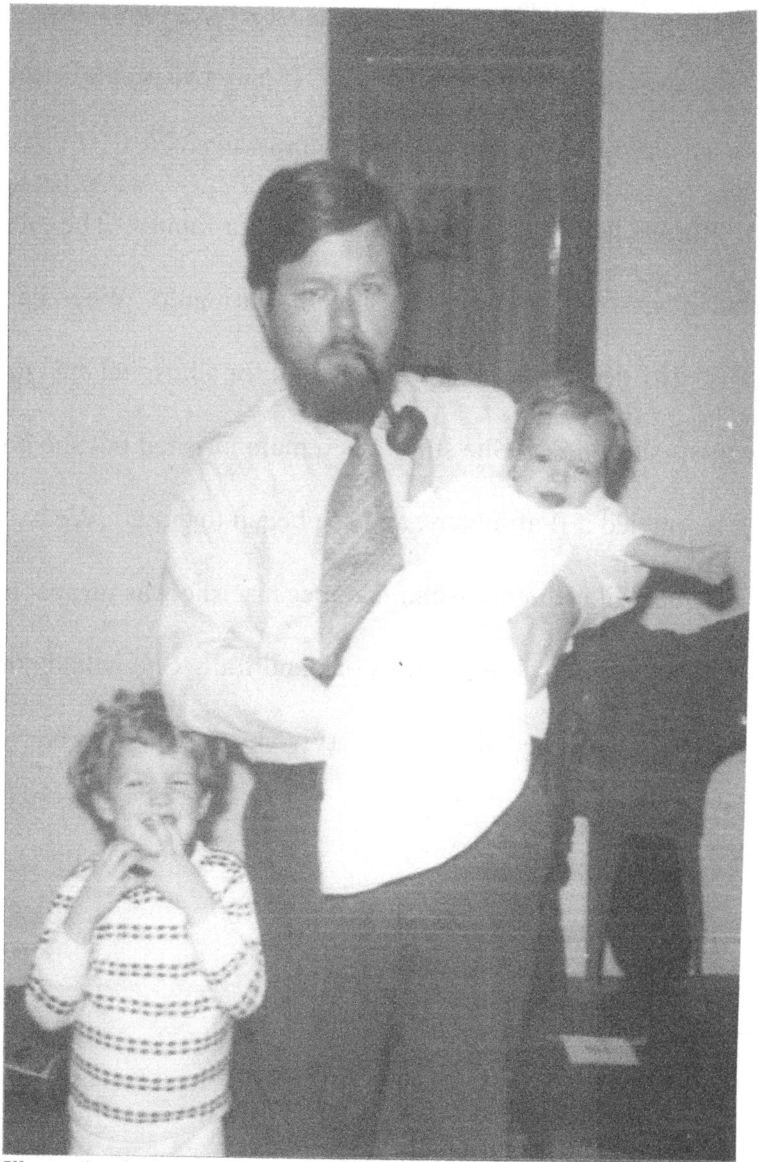

Illustration 2: Aaron, Tony, and Jennifer, winter 1972

Appreciative of each day we had with Jennifer, we led as normal a life as possible. Delighted to be home, we celebrated Christmas with our extended family of brothers and sisters and their children. We lived in a large nineteenth century house a short distance from Richmond, and I invited everyone for Christmas dinner. Cooking a twenty-five pound turkey, everyone came bearing their special dishes. Twenty-two people celebrated with us, not only Christmas but Jennifer's homecoming.

Normal held a different meaning for our family. The infection had abated but was still there, occasionally flaring up. When her fever went over 101 degrees we knew we were in for a hospital stay to get intravenous antibiotics. She still looked malnourished but she no longer resembled a Biafra baby, and she began to crawl. We had been told she would likely never walk. Not because she was incapable of learning but because she was very weak and frail. She would not have the strength to walk, and would not survive long enough or be well enough to learn.

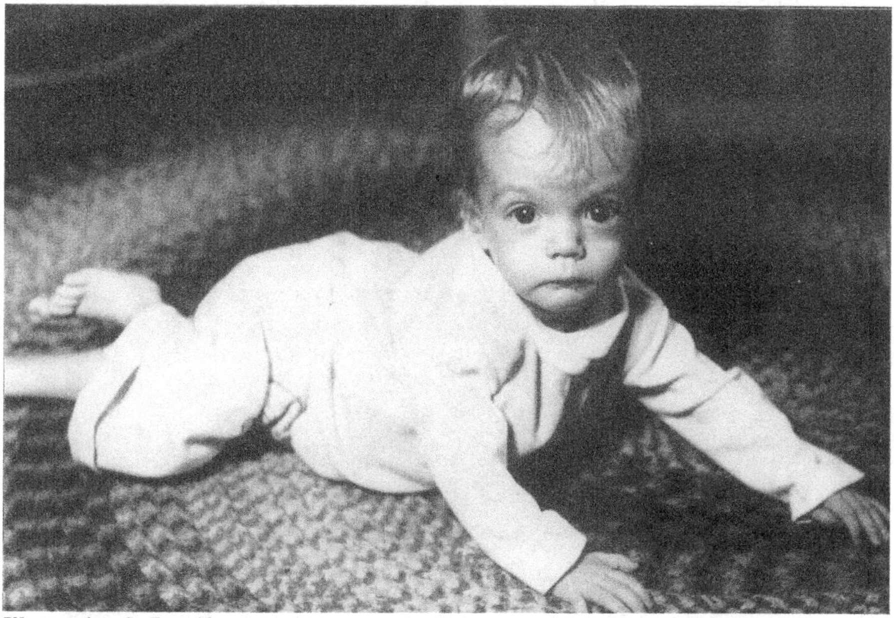

Illustration 3: Jennifer, learning to crawl, 1973

There are memories that stay as fresh as the day they are formed. Our extended family traditionally rented a place on either a river or the ocean for two to three weeks every summer. It was at the river, in a big old rambling house with all the cousins running and playing where one of those memories was made. Crawling across the floor, trying to keep up with her mobile cousins, Jennifer grabbed the side of a chair, pulling up. Without any apparent hesitation, she started walking across the room to her cousins. Sitting at the table talking to my sisters, it did not register. When it did I was speechless. She had done it so effortlessly and with such ease it appeared the most natural thing in the world. So effortless the other adults in the room had a difficult time understanding why I was suddenly reduced to tears. Jennifer, not expected to live beyond the age of eighteen months, was walking.

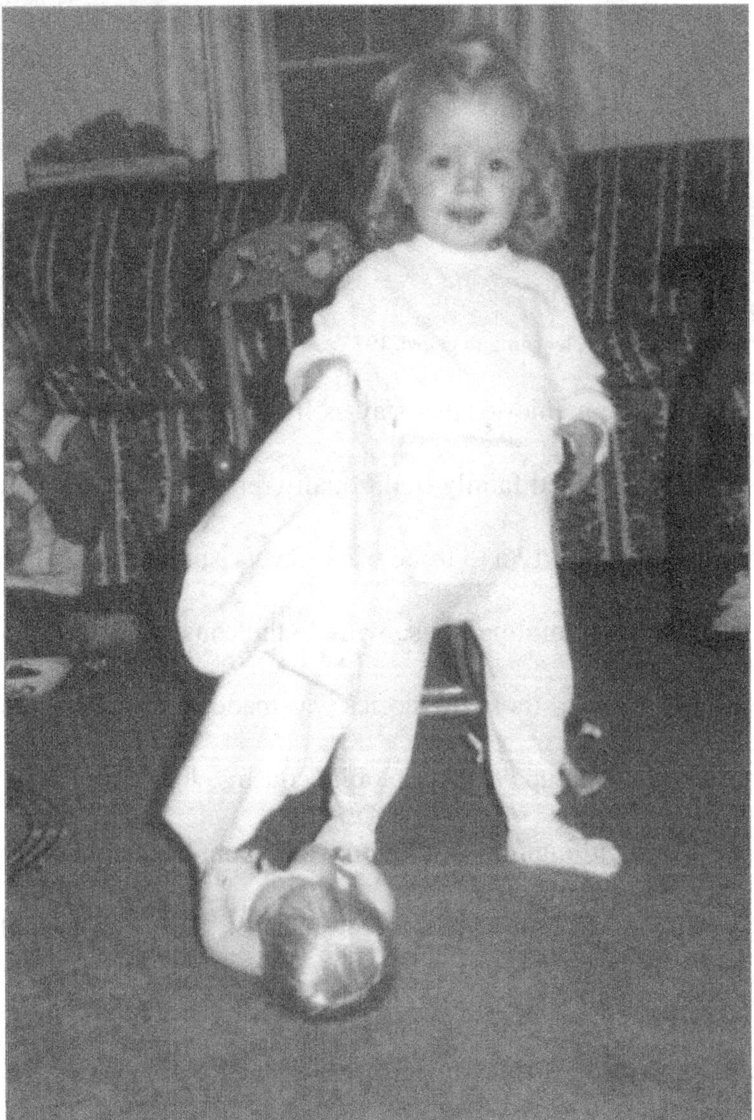

Illustration 4: Jennifer walking, 1974

CHAPTER TWO

NORMALCY, OR THE LACK OF IT

I am in line at the grocery store, Jennifer sitting in the cart facing me and Aaron walking beside me. A young mother pulls into line behind me, smiling at Aaron with his masses of red, cork screw curly hair. Tall for his age, he is shy, and moves closer to Jennifer in the basket. Leaning around to look better at Jennifer, the woman's face hardens into a plastic smile and she steps back. From a distance Jennifer's skin appears olive tone, but it is obvious up close she is severely jaundiced. The woman's reaction is a gut reaction to the unknown: does she have something contagious? Are my children in danger?

Did life become normal for Jennifer and her family once she began to walk? What is normal? Normal was going to birthday parties with her older brother and cousins. Normal was swimming in backyard wading pools on hot summer days. Not normal was having a young mother step back, afraid of what they don't understand. Not normal was the care and effort spent to make sure the bile did not leak from the stoma bag in the wading pool. Not normal was the extended belly and jaundice. Normal was my heartbreak when she was shunned by others, fearful she might be contagious. It was difficult to accept their reactions were normal – they were reacting to something not familiar. Our lives could not be described as normal for a typical young family with two children but we developed our own concept of routine and normalcy. Normal was when the stoma bag stayed in place, when the pen rose drain did not slip out, when infection did not set in.

Normal was Jennifer sitting in her chair eating rainbow sherbet and cake. Unable to property digest the fat in milk, sherbet became her ice cream. Unable to eat regular bread for the same reason, she grew up eating French bread. To this day French bread is a comfort food for Jennifer. What was Jennifer's diet? Low protein and low fat. Lots of chicken and fish. Baked or broiled but never fried. It would be years before Jennifer had butter on her bread, and red meat was totally forbidden. Hamburgers and hot dogs, staples in most children's diets, were not part of her diet. It was not until chicken dogs and turkey burgers became popular did Jennifer enjoy these foods common to most children in the United States. Jennifer's dietary restrictions actually put her ahead of the times. Never allowed fried foods, she never became accustomed to the fried foods so common at most fast food establishments.

How did this affect the rest of the family? In subtle ways it definitely affected the family. Her older brother grew to hate milk and to this day refuses to eat mayonnaise. Where did this come from? Before Jennifer's birth he drank milk like any other two and three year old. Although he does not remember it, I arrived at the conclusion it was from a simple overheard conversation I had with her doctor. What were we talking about? The fact that Jennifer could not drink milk or eat things such as mayonnaise due to the fat content. Sitting on the floor, listening as children will do, Aaron had overheard me talking to her doctor. At the age of three or four how this must have translated to him – milk and products such as mayonnaise were not good for you. If they were bad for Jennifer, why wouldn't they be bad for him. I am sure there were other conversations he must have overheard, other comments and conversations that had an impact upon his view of things. Even my mother, Jennifer and Aaron's grandmother, was affected by Jennifer's diagnosis. She had always enjoyed fried onions and liver, but after Jennifer's birth she told me she could never eat another piece of liver. It had never been a favorite dish of mine, but I certainly felt the same way.

Did these dietary restrictions have an impact upon the family? Not intentionally, although I am sure there were other subtle and not so subtle consequences as was the case with the milk and mayonnaise. I continued to serve beef and a regular diet to the rest of the family, cooking and providing separately for Jennifer as needed. Some changes were easy to make. The Southern fried chicken I grew up eating for Sunday dinners and picnics no longer was a staple of our diet. I baked, baked, and baked some more. Any food Jennifer was allowed to share with us, such as the chicken and fish, was baked, not fried. In this regard it benefited the whole family. As the years went by, I reached a point where I no longer ate beef and eventually stopped cooking it. Chicken and fish became staples in our diet, and if anyone in the family wanted steak they had to cook it themselves. I was glad to buy it but refused to cook it. Most of my extended family members were understanding, although I did get comments about how I was being unfair to the rest of the family, not cooking beef. I could not stand to handle red meat – it reminded me too much of liver. I always took an offering of a vegetarian or poultry dish to family dinners, not expecting others to provide alternatives just for Jennifer. What about spices? In retrospect the family benefited, but no spices were added during cooking to anything Jennifer ate. Food entering her intestine did not have the benefit of bile for digestion, and heavy spices caused stomach aches and cramps. Bile, draining from the stoma, was particularly corrosive to the surrounding skin if she had consumed heavy spices. Eliminating spices was the answer.

Normal was frequent visits to doctors and hospitals. Not only was she a toddler requiring the normal, frequent visits to the doctors, she was paving a path through uncharted territory even the doctors were not familiar with. Should she get the usual immunization shots most toddler's receive? She had defied their expectations, but what did the future hold for her? Would she survive long enough to attend school? If so, would she be well enough to go to school? Aaron was two years older and she would be exposed to the usual childhood illnesses from him. The decision was yes, she did receive them, and suffered no adverse effects from them. The one immunization shot she did not receive, the chicken pox vaccine, was not available at this time. This unknowingly would be a problem later in life, after she received a transplant, and no longer was able to receive live vaccines.

Uncharted waters. That was the perception of the physicians who worked with Jennifer. What to expect when biliary atresia was such a rare condition? What to expect from this blond haired little girl with the big smile who had defied expectations? We had a wonderful group of physicians and surgeons at the Medical College of Virginia, where Jennifer was born. But doctors are just people, like everyone else. Some handled Jennifer better than others. Some, aware of her prognosis, were distant, not allowing themselves to become attached. There was even one who warned me about becoming too attached. Too attached! He was a very good physician, but I was shocked. The attachment and bond is immediate upon the birth of the child. How would you not become too attached?

One physician who handled children with digestive problems such as Jennifer's would return to school to do a residency in anesthesiology. Not only did she handle Jennifer, who as far as we could determine was the only child in the practice with biliary atresia, she also worked with children with cystic fibrosis. An inherited illness, in the 1970s the life expectancy of these children was very poor. She commented to me at the time, when transferring Jennifer's care to another doctor, she found it increasingly difficult to work with children who seldom lived beyond their early years. We missed her greatly as she had empathy for the children we did not see in many of the doctors.

We had picnics, trips to the beach, family get-togethers, and all the activities associated with young children. Other children came over to play, swim, and have birthday parties. The difference was reciprocal activities at the homes of other children. Aaron was invited, but Jennifer was not included unless I was with her. Others were afraid they would not be able to handle the stoma bag, afraid some emergency would occur they would not be able to handle. I understood, but it became increasingly difficult as Jennifer got older and realized she was not included. She and I were both fortunate I had a twin sister living in Richmond who had no qualms about watching Jennifer. Jennifer spent many happy hours with Aaron and her son Chris, only six months older than she, playing and going places together. All of her cousins welcomed her – she was part of the family and in their eyes she was just that – a cousin to laugh and play with. She was good natured and happy – it made no difference to them she had a stoma and had to made frequent trips to the doctors. That was just Jennifer – no different than being blond and blue eyed. She was always welcomed with open arms by my extended family and never made to feel different or out of place.

How did Jennifer's medical condition affect her father's and my relationship? People have asked and I have no answer for them. We both wanted children and were delighted when they were born. This was life. You did what you had to do to manage things. We never felt it impeded us – we were concerned about Jennifer and her well-being. Yes, I was busy, going to the doctors, washing extra laundry due to the drainage form the stoma and taking care of two children. Her father traveled, at times extensively, in his job. Was I upset I had the full time care when he was gone? No, as I knew he would much rather have been home, enjoying the time with the children. In addition we were careful to allow time for the two of us. I was fortunate to live near my twin, as she and my mother both would babysit for us to occasionally get out for dinner or a movie. If there was something special we wanted to do and they were not available, we were, with advance planning, still able to get away for an evening. Teenagers who might have been willing to babysit for two children under five were not an option. They would not have been able to handle Jennifer's stoma , and we did not feel comfortable with their maturity.

Once again our concept of normal or routine was altered. We did not have the routine babysitters but upper level nursing students from the Medical College of Virginia and the two-year nursing program in Richmond. The cost was higher, but we felt comfortable the students, with at least some prior nursing training behind them, could handle Jennifer's stoma and would be more tuned in to any thing that might occur. We were never disappointed, but I wonder today, with all of the threat of lawsuits, if they would be allowed to babysit for someone like Jennifer. Perhaps today with the certification of medical assistants, young mothers in my situation would have an easier time of finding a sitter.

What of family vacations? Were they normal? Once again our view of normal and routine was altered. We did travel to the beach and to the mountains for vacations, but there was a caveat: her physicians had requested we not go any further than a day's ride. Her medical condition was so unique they were concerned there would not be personnel willing or able to help her in an emergency. This was an attitude we would be faced with later when we moved from the comfort of Richmond and the Medical College of Virginia. And it was not the ability but instead the willingness to work with Jennifer that would become an issue. Physicians are people, no different than others, and we would be faced with some who were afraid to handle Jennifer's care. Afraid they would make an incorrect decision and some problem might occur. We were fortunate we lived in Richmond where a short ride would take us to the ocean on the Atlantic coast or the mountains of Virginia.

The Medical College of Virginia (now affiliated with VCU) is a teaching hospital, and we had exceptional physicians and surgeons working with her. Drs. H. M. Lee, Wallace Berman, Gerado Mendez-Picon, and Arnold Salzberg were empathetic, caring, and dedicated to Jennifer's well being. The medical personnel at MCV were not an issue. Instead it was the family physicians not associated with MCV who were charged with her well-baby, routine care. And herein lay the problem. The concept of well-baby care. Jennifer still needed to have a physician to look at her ears, listen to her chest, dispense vaccines, and determine if an episode of fevers was related to her stoma or liver problem or to an illness such as ear infections or colds. She was not the normal toddler going in for routine well-baby care. She was a toddler who had a major liver defect and had defied the odds of the life expectancy for that defect. She needed, in addition to specialized care, routine medical care.

Hers was a condition they had not bargained for in a general family practice – to them she was something they read about in one or two paragraphs in their medical books in school. The text books said their life expectancy was very limited – they felt unsure and unprepared to care for her. Interestingly, the age of the physician did not matter. It seemed to be the personality of the physician and their willingness to handle something new and different. Some of the younger physicians we encountered were as ill-prepared emotionally as some of the older physicians. She was not the routine, normal, textbook child they had been trained to treat in a family practice setting.

CHAPTER THREE

STEPPING OUT

It was not until the late 1980s I was persuaded to eat sushi, and it was only once. I knew it was considered gourmet, and if I had not had Jennifer perhaps I would have loved it. I could not separate my knowledge of some of the potential dangers of eating raw sea food from the succulent taste of the raw tuna. How did Jennifer's birth and subsequent diagnosis affect my desire for sushi? When Jennifer was diagnosed with biliary atresia we were told it was more common in Japan than it was elsewhere. Why? One theory held it may have been caused by hepatitis acquired from eating raw seafood. Raw seafood such as sushi was considered a possibility. I had never eaten raw sea food, but like Aaron's perception of milk and mayonnaise, I am sure the knowledge that raw tuna might be the source of hepatitis made it very unappetizing. There is still today no definitive cause for biliary atresia, but perhaps it was the higher prevalence of biliary atresia in Japan that led to the development of a surgical procedure offered to newborns born with biliary atresia today.

Developed by Dr. Moria Kasai in 1951, at the time of Jennifer's birth in 1972 it was not an option offered to Jennifer. Named after Dr. Kasai, the procedure is also called an hepatoportoenterostomy procedure[iv]. We were told in 1972 the Kasai procedure was considered an experimental surgery and it was not available in the United States. It was listed as an option just as the option of pediatric transplant had been offered to Jennifer. As was the case with the transplant, we were not willing for Jennifer to be a guinea pig It was experimental and our option was to travel to Japan to see about the procedure. It's difficult for people today to envision but in 1972 the Internet was not available. What medical information available to the general population was either directly from physicians and medical personnel or from research done by the patient or their family. How did they accomplish this research? By sitting in the libraries of university medical centers. By calling hospitals who might have any information that applied to a patient such as Jennifer. Remember, pediatric liver transplantation was considered an experimental surgery. In addition the tests used today to diagnose biliary atresia are more sophisticated than they were in 1972. It was not until Jennifer was almost a month old was she diagnosed. Today, the Kasai procedure is performed on babies diagnosed with biliary atresia, and the success is greatest when it is done before the infant is one month old.

To perform the Kasai procedure, surgeons first carefully remove the damaged ducts outside of the liver. They use a small segment of the patient's own intestine to replace the ducts at the spot where bile is expected to drain. This segment not only connects to the liver, but also connects to the rest of the intestine. The Y-shaped passageway formed by the Kasai procedure allows bile to flow from the liver into the intestine.

Small, Jennifer had continued to gain weight slowly. But at the age of three and a half it was obvious she had come to a standstill. Bile is necessary in the intestine to digest food and the bile had continued to flow out the stoma. Her physicians recommended the Kasai procedure, and we were forced to decide whether the risk was worth it. She had done so well, relatively speaking, it was a difficult decision to make. But she had reached a plateau – we did not want her to slide down the other side. Something had to be done to increase the nutrients her body was able to digest.

What would become of the stoma she had dealt with since shortly after birth? Much to our disappointment they decided she needed to maintain the stoma to help relieve pressure on the liver. They would perform the Kasai procedure, which would help direct bile to her intestine, but the stoma would remain. Jennifer had no recollection of life without the stoma, but we were disappointed. It had become increasingly difficult to maintain a clean environment for Jennifer as she grew. The position of the stoma made it difficult to maintain bags over the site, and the bile seemed to be corrosive to any seal we tried on the bag. We often resorted to 4 x 4 bandages instead of the bags to trap the bile but they were not effective. If Jennifer ate or drank any significant amount of food the bile would pour out of the stoma and it would be necessary to change the bags or bandages as well as her clothes. Bile is corrosive to the skin and we were constantly trying to prevent her skin from breaking down around the stoma. If we used anything such as petroleum jelly the bag would not adhere to the skin at all, but if the bile drained out of the stoma bag onto her skin it not only created an unseemly yellow wetness on her clothing but irritated the skin. It was a constant battle and a no-win situation, one which would be a problem for years.

Jennifer came through the Kasai procedure with flying colors. The stoma was still in place, but some bile was entering the intestines and helping with digestion. She would never grow by leaps and bounds but she was growing and gaining weight at a constant rate. The Kasai would help Jennifer to grow but it was unable to provide the benefit it provides to some of the children born with biliary atresia today. Bile is essential for digestion of food, but if it remains in the liver it eventually destroys the cells of the liver, causing cirrhosis. A percentage of the children undergoing the Kasai before the age of one month will maintain enough normal liver function and will never have to undergo a transplant. This was not the case with Jennifer, as the cirrhosis is cumulative, and at the age of three her liver was being destroyed. Was the surgery worth it? Yes, as it enabled her to grow and reduced some of the flow of bile backing up into the liver. But it was not a cure and her prognosis remained the same.

Jennifer had reached one of her "plateau periods." These were periods we would look back upon and realize they were our family's version of normal. There were still infections to combat, mad rushes to the hospital to receive intravenous antibiotics, and there were still crises, but we had our own version of normal and routine. Routine did not mean the same to us as it did to most, and something as common as the flu could cause chaos in our normal life.

It is midnight, and instead of racing down Broad Street to MCV I am going west, in a rush to get home from MCV. The year was 1976, and Jennifer was four. Thirty-four years later the country is faced with a similar potential threat but almost no one remembers 1976. Jennifer had become ill, increasingly lethargic and feverish, and we knew she needed to be seen at MCV. Her physician was alarmed at how quickly she had deteriorated and how unresponsive she was, and she was immediately hospitalized. The flu, and she was terribly ill. How had this happened so quickly? The day before she had been fine.

A variant of the seasonal flu had been identified, and the country was in a panic. Was this the flu, dubbed the swine flu, everyone was so terrified of? None of us had been vaccinated, and it might have been the seasonal variety of the flu. Her father had become ill a few days before and we had assumed it was the usual flu. I had spent two hours getting Jennifer settled into the hospital, and had not been able to get an answer when I called home. Why was the phone not answered? It was midnight, and I was in a rush to get home, check on Tony and Aaron, and return to the hospital to be with my sick little girl.

Walking into the house it was quiet – too quiet. The dining room was in disarray, chairs facing backwards from the table with a rope interloped in between the backing of the Queen Anne chairs. Walking quickly into Aaron's bedroom, I found him asleep on his bed, in his pajamas, but no answer from his father. Passing the bathroom I saw water spilling slowly over the side of the tub onto the floor. Panicked, I rushed to our bedroom, finding Jennifer's father under piles of blankets, shivering, and unable to respond to my questions. Burning up, he had a fever of 105 degrees. Whatever Jennifer and he had was very dangerous. Stripping the blankets off the bed and forcing him to remove his shirt I washed him down with wet cloths, bringing his fever down to a manageable level. He had no memory of the time I had been gone with Jennifer, and had felt so badly he had not even taken any aspirin or Tylenol before lying down. Aaron had taken care of himself, and I was horrified.

I was desperate to get back to the hospital to Jennifer – I had no idea how she was and had never left her in the hospital by herself when she was so ill. Persuading Tony to get into the shower, his temperature was finally close to normal. Stripping the bed of all but one light blanket, I set a supply of water beside the bed and another dose of aspirin in a cup. My mother, living 20 miles away, was waiting for Aaron. She would watch him so I could go back to the hospital and have the freedom to return home to check on Tony. Aaron and I drove to his grandmother Mimi's house at three in the morning. So far he was well, and she would watch him while I went back to check on Tony and to the hospital. What had occurred while I was gone? Tony had suddenly become ill, lying down on the bed, and Aaron had decided to make a fence with the rope around the dining room table. Fixing himself a peanut butter sandwich for dinner, he had them drawn his own bath and gotten ready for bed, but had forgotten to turn the water off. I was impressed yet saddened he had to take care of himself. Emergencies happen in all families, but they were more frequent in our family. And what was this flu? Was is the swine flu of 1976? We would never know but considered ourselves lucky to have survived it. Did we get the vaccine they were giving out at the time? No, none of us had been inoculated, and in retrospect we were very glad.

Our intention with Jennifer was to have her lead as normal a life as possible. She had few limitations other than her diet and the limitations placed on her by outsiders who did not understand or were afraid of her condition. What do many three year olds do? If they have not been in daycare they frequently experience their first school setting. We were fortunate there was a pre-school across the street from our home in Richmond. The owner was kind and understanding, and not afraid of Jennifer's condition. She agreed to have Jennifer enroll in the program two mornings a week, and Jennifer loved it. Aaron was in Kindergarten and in her mind she was now a big girl, going to school like Aaron. Were there restrictions placed on Jennifer by the owner? None, except the request I let her know if I was going to be away from home during those periods and to leave an emergency phone number. Jennifer was stepping out for the first time. It was a momentous day for her and for me.

CHAPTER FOUR

INTO THE UNKNOWN
(Do cows moo ALL night?)

Big changes were in store, for all of the family. Tony had decided to return to graduate school, and we were leaving behind everything that was comfortable and routine. We were moving to the mountains of Virginia from the City of Richmond. Christiansburg, VA, seven miles from the Virginia Tech Campus in Blacksburg, would be our home for the next four years. No longer would we be living in a fairly large, vibrant city with a well-known and respected Medical Center with the support of extended family but instead would be living in a new community outside the small college town of Blacksburg. No longer would we hear the traffic of a well traveled street outside the windows, but instead the mooing of the cows in the pasture down the street. Stray cats would not be a problem – there were few, largely because of the occasional mountain lion that would appear on the deck of the back of our home or the black bear we would occasionally see at dusk as we drove home.

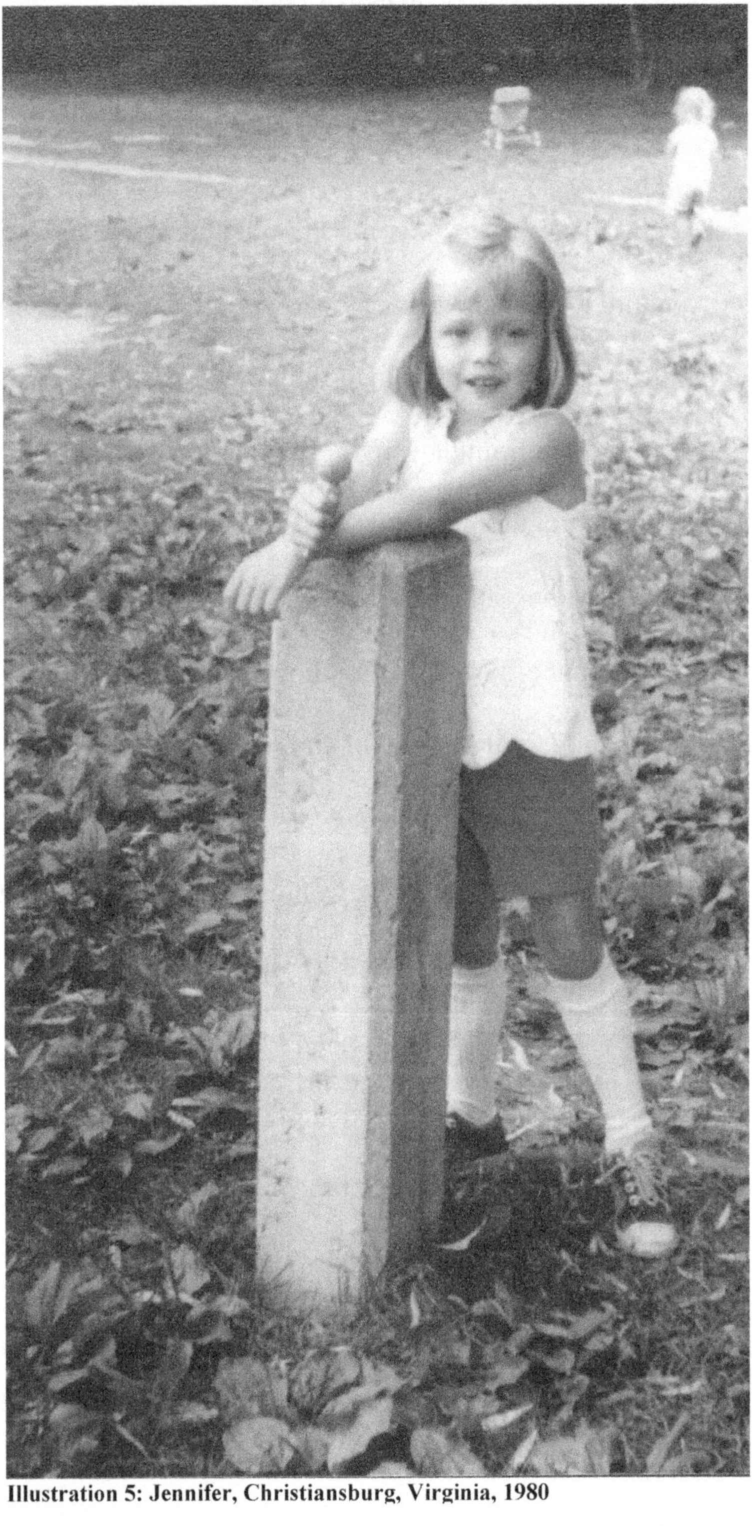

Illustration 5: Jennifer, Christiansburg, Virginia, 1980

Five and almost eight, it was an adventure for Jennifer and Aaron, and it was here Jennifer would start public school. We had checked on the school system and it was considered exceptional – many of the teachers were spouses of professors from Tech. What we had not counted on was the difficulty in identifying medical personnel to take charge of Jennifer's routine care. We had assumed we would easily identify a pediatrician or family practice doctor , but that was not to be the case. Biliary atresia? A child five years old with a chronic liver condition they had only read about in their medical textbooks, and one who was in uncharted waters? The pool of physicians was not extensive in such a small community, but we were finally able to locate a physician who agreed to handle Jennifer's care. Richmond was only six hours away by car, and we knew if necessary she could be flown to Richmond in an emergency. It was the routine care of colds and sore throats we needed help with. It was not until later, when we did face an emergency and were living in Christiansburg that I realized truly how fortunate we had been to find him. A two man practice, the older physician in the group had been opposed to allowing Jennifer to become a patient. It was only with assurances from the young physician on the team that he would assume responsibility would the senior member of the practice agree to take her on as a patient.

The Kasai procedure had helped, and Jennifer remained well. We were on another plateau, but we never knew when it would end. She had wonderful teachers at school – some of the best she would face in the public school setting. They were understanding and not demanding of my time, although I made sure to be available in case she needed a clothing change. Cell phones were still in the future for everyday use – I made sure to have phone numbers available to the school. She was very independent, and with multiple changes of clothing kept at school, she often did not even need to call me if the bile had soaked through her clothing. She changed her clothes herself, often without the help of teachers. She was older, and made a point of not eating foods she knew would irritate her, or to drink so much she would drain too much. She would wait to do that after school, drinking copious quantities of liquids. She never seemed to be able to get enough to drink, but when she did large amounts of bile would come pouring out of her stoma.

Our time in Christiansburg is remembered with fondness by all of us. Jennifer loved school, riding the bus everyday with Aaron, and made numerous friends. I made a point of volunteering often at school, for more than one reason. In addition to spending time with the children, it gave me an opportunity to assure the teachers I would be available and was accessible. I became the leader of Jennifer's Brownie Troop. Not something I had thought about doing, I instinctively knew it would be better. We would not face the issue of other mothers' fear of Jennifer's problem. I would be in constant attendance when planned activities took place, and there would be no question of Jennifer being excluded.

Christiansburg is in the mountains, and our house was at the bottom of a steep hill. So steep that in the snows of winter we put sandbags in the trunk of our old car to give it the added traction to get to the top of the hill. Jennifer's independence and determination have always been her hallmarks, but sometimes it terrified me.

At the age of six she begged for a bike, and we finally relented, realizing it would be better if we taught her to ride instead of having her go to a friend's house and get injured learning. Little did we know that would not even be enough for Jennifer. On a cold, clear day after Christmas, Aaron and Jennifer were outside, bundled up against the cold that sometimes would dip below 0° Fahrenheit. Looking out the window, I saw a streak of blond hair flying by, weaving all over the road. Terrified, I dashed out the door. She had no concept of riding the bike and no knowledge of applying the brakes. By the time I was out the door she was at the end of the street, at the bottom of a steep hill, bike and Jennifer lying on the ground. Running down the street, I was sure I would find her seriously injured. We had been told she was to play no contact sports due to the danger of injury to the spleen, liver, or stoma, and there she was, lying on the ground, bike beside her.

Miraculously, she was uninjured except for a skinned knee and elbow. She later told me she knew she was going too fast, and had steered towards the fence to stop the bike. Her reaction? "Mommy, I know how to ride now. I can go places with Aaron!" Jennifer's determination to just be another one of the kids became legendary as she grew older. Can this determination be taught or is it inborn? The family has always laughed, as Jennifer has always reminded the family of her grandmother Mimi, who over her lifetime flew in the face of opposition many times, determined to not let her gender affect what she wanted to accomplish in life.

Trooper and helicopter pilot on the Governor's detail. Quiet and restrained, he was the epitome of a State Trooper. Retired from the military, he'd flown helicopters in Vietnam and had survived a number of crashes. Climbing in the back of the car, I had no idea what lay ahead. What was wrong with Jennifer? Would we make it to the hospital in time? Tony told me to keep applying gentle pressure on her abdomen, and the flow of blood had diminished. My hands were sticky with Jennifer' blood, and I felt the dampness of her blood soaked clothes against my skin. My last sign of Tony and Aaron was as they stood on the porch, Tony washing the blood off the porch.

Lights flashing, I paid little attention to our speed. Frustrated and angry people were not pulling to the side of the road, ignoring the flashing lights. What did the Trooper do? He straddled the middle of the road, forcing the cars to the side of the road. It was usually less than half an hour to the hospital, and we made the trip in record time. Medical personnel waited for us at the emergency entrance and rushed Jennifer into an examining room.

And … nothing. There was no sign of bleeding. Only the blood soaked clothes and my soaked hands and clothes. Blood work confirmed she had lost a large quantity of blood. Her hematocrit was extremely low and she needed to be transfused, but where did the blood come from? Admitted to the hospital, she needed at least two units of blood.

Weak and exhausted, Jennifer slept as I dozed in a chair beside her bed. The hospital was small but very new and went out of its way to make families comfortable. We would stay the night and make plans for a visit to MCV when the offices opened the next day. They would need to evaluate her and determine what had happened.

Waking in the middle of the night, I leaned over the bed to give Jennifer a kiss. She was ice cold. Turning the light on to look for extra blankets, I stared at her bed. Red. Everything was red. The sheets, the edges of the pillow under Jennifer, and the blanket on top of her. And Jennifer was a pale as the sheets should have been. Terrified, I ran to the door, calling for the nurse instead of pushing the call button. Rushing into the room they pulled the blankets and sheet off Jennifer, trying to determine where the blood was coming from. Whatever had caused her to bleed had stopped. Stripping the bed, the bed linens were placed in the corner of the room. The nurse in charge said unless she had them to show the doctor he would never believe the quantity of blood she had lost. Where was the blood coming from?

We had not slid from our plateau – we had taken a dive off the side of it, into an unknown abyss.

Christiansburg is in a valley, and the weather can be very mercurial. Violent summer storms sweep through the valley, producing spectacular displays of lightening. At times a dense, moist fog rolls in heavy and thick, making it almost impossible to see a hand held in front of your face. Thick fog had settled into the valley when the sun came up, and we knew they would not be able to fly Jennifer to Richmond as they planned after her bleeding episode the night before. Jennifer's physician, the young doctor who had been so willing to take Jennifer as a member of the practice, was out-of-town. His partner, older and reluctant to handle a problem such as Jennifer's, was on call that weekend. I had not realized how difficult he found it to work with Jennifer until we were getting into the ambulance. After wishing us a good trip, he asked when we were moving. We had no plans to move anytime soon and I was not sure why he was asking, I repeated his question. "When are we moving?"

His response? "Yes, when are you moving where there is a large medical center?"

It would be another year before we were ready to leave, and at that moment that was the furthest thought from my mind. But it was clear the physician was anxious to have us leave town.

Tony met us at the hospital in Christiansburg, and he later said he thought that would be last time he would ever see Jennifer. Lights flashing, we were racing down the mountains to Richmond and the doctors at MCV.

Jennifer, a nurse, and I were riding in the back of the ambulance when I asked the driver his name. "Speedy is what they call me." As I looked out the window the landscape was a blur, but it was not until we reached Richmond did I realize how fast we must have been traveling. Normally a six hour trip from Christiansburg to Richmond, we had made it in four. Speedy was his name, and he lived up to his reputation.

Jennifer was getting transfused, and there had been no sign of additional bleeding. Even in the worst situations there is sometimes a bit of humor. They were pumping Jennifer full of fluids, giving her a saline solution when she was not getting a unit of blood. What happens to all this fluid? She had to urinate. About an hour into the trip the nurse and I realized we had neglected to bring a container to put the urine in and the bedpan was quickly filling. Speedy, besides being one of the all time fastest and best ambulance drivers, had an answer for everything. Pulling to a screeching halt beside the mountain, he jumped out with the bedpan, throwing the contents against the mountainside. We laughed when we thought about the bob cats and other animals. Would they think a human had been staking out territory?

And what happened once we got into Richmond? We ran into a traffic jam. The two hours shaved off the trip by Speedy were spent sitting in traffic, slowly making our way to MCV. Emergency room personnel had been alerted to our arrival, but here we were, sitting in traffic. Jennifer slept, and the nurse, Speedy and I were grateful there were no signs of additional bleeding.

Finally arriving at MCV, Jennifer was examined and admitted to the hospital. Her physician could not find the source of any bleeding, and the nurse and I both had the uncomfortable feeling they questioned what had occurred. MCV and Richmond were home to Jennifer and to me. We had continued to make regular trips to Richmond to visit family and for Jennifer to be seen by the specialists at MCV. It was our comfort zone. But we had the distinct impression they questioned the sequence of events – what they could not see they were having trouble believing. That would dramatically change, and I was to learn doctors do get angry and upset, and yes, sometimes they do yell.

Twelve hours later there was still no sign of bleeding, and Jennifer had been allowed to go to the playroom on the pediatric floor. Staffed by full-time personnel, parents were not allowed to stay in the playroom. MCV is a teaching hospital, and there are many children who are in the hospital for an extended period of time. If they are school age, there are visiting teachers who work with the children. Sitting in her room, I saw Jennifer walking down the hall towards me, her hand on the wall. Going to meet her, she collapsed in my arms. No crying, no signs of discomfort. Carrying her to her bed, I looked at her gown. The bag covering the stoma was bulging, and I could see through the gown it was not the normal color of bile but was a dark, almost black color. Blood, and the stoma bag was full. Jennifer was extremely weak, and I was afraid to walk away from the bed. Here I was again, rushing to the door, calling for the nurse. What was going on?

Lifting up her gown, the nurse told me not to leave her and rushed out the room. Within a few minutes Jennifer's room became Grand Central Station. Every doctor on staff who had seen her before was crowded into the room, as well as two nurses, one pushing the crash cart into the room. No one knew what was going on and they had coded Jennifer, expecting the worst. How many doctors? To this day I don't know, but there were a lot of starched white coats standing around the bed. What were they doing? They were loudly arguing with one another. Yelling would be a more accurate description. Whose fault was this? What was going on? I was seeing emotions I had not see in her physicians before, reminding me they are just human. Cooler heads prevailed, and they stepped into the hall to continue their discussion. I appreciated their wisdom – it would not have helped Jennifer or me to be reminded they knew no more about what was going on than we did.

Jennifer was unique. She had defied expectations all her life, and many times she and the doctors were swimming in uncharted territory. This proved to be the case again, and what presented so dramatically and was indeed life threatening proved to be relatively simple to repair. Taking her into surgery, her doctors needed to determine the source of bleeding. What was it? Within an hour her surgeon was out of the operating room, smiling and relieved. Due to the enlargement of the spleen and liver and the pressure from the fluid on her abdomen, varices had formed around the stoma. The blood was an arterial pumper at the stoma orifice. It had ruptured, and the blood was pumped out when she moved around. That is why pressure applied to the abdomen had stopped the bleeding. They ligated the varices and the problem was taken care of. A simple fix for a problem that could have been deadly. Jennifer had once again been through uncharted waters, emerging on the other side of the lake.

CHAPTER FIVE

FROM THE MOUNTAINS TO THE OCEAN

(No more cows but lots of fish)

Jennifer's doctor was getting his wish – we were leaving Christiansburg. Down from the mountains and to the ocean – no more cows but lots of fish! Tony had finished his doctorate at Tech and we were moving to Massachusetts. Accepting a year-long position working in Boston, we rented a house in Lexington. We would be living in a small town where we could walk to stores and activities, and we were excited about getting to sight see around the Boston area. The downside was the change of medical personnel. Once again we were going to have to change doctors. Not only would we need to identify a family physician, but we needed to establish contact with a teaching hospital. Boston was twice the distance to MCV as Christiansburg and Jennifer needed someone closer. Boston is renowned for its teaching institutions, and we were confident we'd have no problem.

We were wrong, and it had nothing to do with the high quality of the medical care available in Boston. It was here, in one of Boston's leading medical institutions, we made the decision "if it works, don't change it." Children were still not surviving who were born with biliary atresia, and Jennifer was nine years old. Pediatric transplant surgery was still in its infancy. The Kasai procedure, which Jennifer had at the age of three, was extending the life of newborns born with biliary atresia, but their prognosis was still bleak. We were confronted by a team of physicians whose main thrust was "we'd never have done this, we'd never do that" when it came to Jennifer's care. They were absolutely negative in their assessment of Jennifer's care at MCV. "Look at her, she survived. They must have done something right!" was my response. Physicians, with their life and death decisions, have their share of hubris. They would not be able to make the decisions they are forced to make unless they did, but again, as when she was a newborn, we were being told their opinions and decisions were supreme. They wanted to perform surgeries we did not feel comfortable with and change medications we felt had worked for Jennifer. What was our response?

The train. Jennifer and I decided we would continue her care at MCV. It was an easy train ride from Boston to Richmond, and we made the trip every few months to return to MCV and their care. It became an adventure for us, and we had multiple family members to stay with in Richmond. She and I, and sometimes Aaron, would reserve sleepers and make the trip to Richmond. If an emergency arose we planned on flying her to Richmond once she was stabilized. We were not willing to change what had worked for Jennifer. This would not be the last time Jennifer would be faced with physicians who wanted to change what had worked for her, and it would not be the last time she said no.

CHAPTER SIX

MEMORIES – JENNIFER SPEAKS

I have wonderful memories of our time in Christiansburg. I had a friend, a girl my age, who lived next door to us, and we were very close. Looking back, I appreciate her mother and father even more today. I did not think about it when I was in Kindergarten, but I realize today how understanding and accepting they were. Many of the other parents were not. I loved riding the school bus with Aaron and going to school, but it was at school I first faced ostentation, avoidance, and bullying by other children and their parents.

The exterior drain was horrible. I had to watch everything I ate and drank. Something too salty or spicy, I would drain excessively and the drainage would burn the skin around the stoma. When the surgeons located the stoma site when I was a new born they must not have allowed for growth, or perhaps the increased size of my stomach and abdomen was the problem. An ostomy bag would never stay in place and I usually had sterile pads over it. The bile was corrosive to my skin, and the skin would become raw and red and burn horribly.

It was a Catch 22 situation. If I drank too much I would drain, but I was thirsty all the time. When we went to the store I never got a small drink – I would get the largest cup they sold and finish it before anyone else finished their drink. The seal around the bag would leak, and we'd have to put sterile pads over the drain. The bile gushed out, soaking my clothes.

We kept a change of clothing at school for me – multiple changes of clothing. The teachers were nice, but they didn't want to touch the bile soaked clothes and I was responsible for changing my clothes if the school nurse was not there. That is a big responsibility for a Kindergarten student. At times it was so bad Mom would have to pick me up at school as I would not stop draining. This meant more time missed from school, and a lot of embarrassment. The other children did not understand what was happening and thought I had wet myself. It drained so much it would gush out, go around my back, and down my shorts or pants. The kids laughed and made fun of me. How could a five or six year old explain something like that?

It wasn't only the bile draining they made fun of – my stomach was big because of the fluid accumulating. My eyes were yellow, or jaundiced, and some of the kids in the class would make fun of me and bully me. I was called yellow eyes, yellow girl, and alien girl – lots of hurtful names. It just got worse as I got older – the kids were even meaner.

No one wanted to work with me in group activities so I always worked by myself. As I got older gym class was a nightmare as no one wanted me on their team, even in just passing a ball around. To this day I don't know why the teachers didn't intervene and make them include me. It wasn't so bad in Kindergarten and first grade, but later I would spend most of my time by myself. I would jump rope, play basketball by myself, or just sit and read in the corner. Maybe I should be thankful somewhat as it taught me at an early age to be independent and self sufficient and I grew to love reading. Reading was where I could escape into another world – someplace where people were not calling me names or making fun of me. I decided I would never treat other people like they treated me. I know today it was ignorance on their part, but to a five or six year old it can be devastating.

And the adults? I understand today where the children got their attitude. I had a few girl friends I played with, but most parents would not invite me over. I am sure the leaking bile offended and frightened them. On one hand I can understand, but for a child it is difficult to be excluded. Not just excluded, but avoided. They avoided me, avoided looking at me except when my back was turned. Not only was I prevented from playing any contact sports due to the risk of injury, I was at times prevented from even going onto the playing field. They were worried about injuries and liability and would not listen when my parents tried to explain that was not an issue. They were not going to hold anyone liable for any unforeseen event – I was allowed to have as normal a childhood at home as much as possible. Today I can't imagine anyone would be able to deny me the opportunity to go onto a public playing field, funded by public money. I learned later it became a real issue when we lived in Massachusetts. My parents shielded me from negative reactions and attitudes as much as possible. This would become more difficult as I grew older and spent more time in activities away from home.

After a year in Lexington, Massachusetts, we were on the move again – back to our home state of Virginia. My Dad was going to be working at the Northern Virginia Campus of Virginia Tech, and we settled into a new house in a suburb of Fairfax. It was in Fairfax, walking home from school in the fourth grade, I had a particularly nasty experience.

You read stories in the papers about children attacking and hurting other children, apparently without remorse. As I grew older, into my late elementary and middle school years, I also faced this. I always had friends, but for some children, verbally abusing me was not enough. I was ten years old. I had made friends although I was always suspect of other children's intentions – I had been bullied and made fun of too often. Walking home from school one day I was attacked and beaten – not by the wild boys in the class but by one of the girls. We had been friends at one time and I never understood what happened and why she turned on me. Twice my size, I never understood why she disliked me so much. I was not severely injured but it was clear when I walked into the house after school something had happened. And what was the reaction of the school? They found it hard to believe that particular girl would do anything violent and questioned what had really happened. The incident was ignored and pushed under the carpet – I don't think anyone ever believed what had happened. With all the awareness programs against bullying today I am hoping they would be more receptive and understanding. Any child, male or female, is in danger of being bullied and it is a horrible experience.

I don't remember being bitter. That is more of an adult reaction. I was hurt and embarrassed. I had a wonderful relationship with Aaron and my cousin Chris, who is only six months older than I am. They included me in all of their activities – riding bikes, playing with Star Wars figures, going to movies. I was very close to my three older female cousins, Lela, Lisa and Stephanie, who treated me like a younger sister and member of their family. I had a wonderful relationship with all my cousins. I am not sure any of them ever viewed me as different – they had never known me any differently. They were not ashamed or embarrassed by me, and Aaron and Chris would prevent anyone saying anything mean or negative about me, chasing them down the street. Aaron protected me at school and the other children knew better than to be mean when he was anywhere nearby. It was the times when he was not around I was most in danger.

CHAPTER SEVEN

LETTING GO – CAMP HOLIDAY TRAILS

We were on the move again, back to Virginia. No more train rides from Boston to Richmond to see Jennifer's physicians at MCV. Tony had accepted a job at the Northern Virginia Campus of Virginia Tech, and we were only two hours away from MCV. We enjoyed our year in Boston and all it had to offer, but we were delighted to get back to Virginia. Closer to family and MCV, six weeks of snow on the ground in the Boston area had made us appreciative of the milder climate of Virginia. The month of May in Virginia is beautiful, and we were glad to be on our way home.

We were on another plateau, and Jennifer was doing well. Determined to be just another kid, she was furious at the age of nine to not be allowed to go away to camp as her brother and cousins did each summer. They came home talking about their friends, the canoeing and horseback riding, the trains and airplanes they rode to get to their camps. Why couldn't she go away to camp? I couldn't imagine her going away to some place where she was an unknown. I had taken care of her on a daily basis for nine years – how would she manage without my supervision and help? How could she participate in camp activities when some people denied her the opportunity to attend events on public property?

Showing her trademark of determination and independence, she was the one who buttonholed her doctor at MCV and demanded an answer. “Why can't I go? I do everything all the other kids do.” She was right, but the difference was either her father or I were with her when she participated in activities such as horseback riding or swimming. One of us was with her in case she ran into problems or did not feel well. Who would look after her as well as we did? She had achieved so much more than was ever expected but we had always been there for her.

I was surprised when we were told there was such a place – a camp where children with chronic health needs had the opportunity to stay overnight and experience all the activities most children take for granted. Camp Holiday Trails, nestled in a beautiful setting just outside Charlottesville, Virginia, was staffed by nurses and medical students from The University of Virginia. There was tubing down the James River, horseback riding, sleeping in cabins, and swimming in the pools, lakes, and rivers in the area. Would they accept Jennifer as a camper? Jennifer was unique – most biliary atresia patients did not do as well as Jennifer. Her physician at MCV was unsure, but felt confident enough to have mentioned it to us. Camp Holiday Trails opened in 1976 – just five years before. What types of chronic illnesses were they familiar with? Again, there was no Internet available. We would have to wait to receive literature and the application in the mail, but her physician assured us he would recommend Jennifer as a camper.

Would I be able to let her go? It would be very difficult, but I knew if they accepted her I would have to agree. Our goal had always been to let her lead as normal a life as possible. How could I deny her the opportunity? I would have to trust the camp personnel's judgment – if they felt they could handle the biliary atresia – she deserved the opportunity to experience what her brother and cousins had experienced.

Jennifer, accepted as a camper at Camp Holiday Trails for a two-week session, was beside herself with excitement. We went shopping for everything on her list, including a trunk to take to camp with her all her possessions. The night before her departure to Camp Jennifer packed and repacked her trunk to make sure she had everything she wanted and needed. Favorite books, mementos from home, and plenty of writing paper with pre-stamped envelopes. She would not be allowed to call home nor we to call her unless there was an emergency – we would communicate by mail. Tony sat on the floor with Jennifer and showed her how to roll her clothing in the trunk to make more space – just as he had done when he went to boot camp for the Coast Guard. It was very difficult for both of us to let her go.

It was the middle of June, and we were riding into the hills of Virginia to Charlottesville. Who in Virginia has not heard of UVA – or as many call it "THE University." Considered one of the premier universities on the East Coast, it was at the top of the list of many college-bound graduating seniors. The medical school was well respected – how could we say no to this experience for Jennifer when the staff appeared to be so competent and confident?

Tucked away, along a dirt road outside of Charlottesville, the Camp was beautiful. A huge dining hall overlooked the woods – the hills looked awfully steep from where I stood. Chris and Aaron had ridden with us to Charlottesville, and both wanted to stay at camp with Jennifer. They had been going to camp themselves for two years, but they did not want to go home without Jennifer. There were bunks for the campers, a large swimming pool, and a pristine and well stocked medical infirmary where the nurses and medical students worked in shifts. We saw the tubes she would float down the James River on and my heart was in my mouth. Float down the River? And I would not be there beside her? She knew how to swim, but had never done anything like tubing before. We walked the grounds with Jennifer, and then settled her into her cabin. It was time to go. Would I be able to talk to her that night to make sure she was OK? No, but I would be able to call the infirmary to check on her. They knew, after the initial excitement, there would be homesickness and found it was better if the campers did not talk to anyone from home for the first few days.

How difficult it was to drive back to Northern Virginia without Jennifer, knowing I would not be able to talk with her. It would be at least three days before I got a letter from her. How was I to know whether she was really feeling well? Were they capable of taking care of her as I did at home? It was a lonely house when we arrived home, and I was glad Chris was visiting to keep Aaron occupied.

Did it go well? An unqualified yes is the answer. She was homesick but did not admit to it in her letters. Her letters were filled with the excitement of making new friends, sitting in front of campfires at night, and all the activities they had scheduled for the campers. She had taken a major step towards independence. Little did I know within two years she would not only go to camp but would take the train to and from Charlottesville by herself, lugging her trunk off and on the train when there was no one to help. Eventually she would be gone for almost five weeks each summer, choosing to stay at camp for three weeks and stopping by Richmond on the way home for two weeks after camp to spend time with her Grandmother Mimi and visit cousins in Richmond. Many healthy children never leave home to go away to camp or visit relatives by themselves, but Jennifer dove in, determined to be "one of the kids."

CHAPTER EIGHT

WHEN PIGS FLY/STOP THE LAUGHTER

Jennifer was still sitting on the plateau. There were the ever present mini-emergencies of trips to the doctors and hospital for visits and exams, but things were as normal as they were ever going to be. She still had the stoma, and that was still a messy situation for Jennifer. She had learned better how to handle it herself, but she was still faced with the ridicule and teasing from other children. Her physicians had decided the stoma had served its purpose and advised us to talk to Jennifer about surgery to shut it off.

But fate seemed to continually hit us broadside, and before this occurred there was a catastrophic public health crisis in the country. The blood supply of the country was contaminated, and she would need multiple units of blood to have the surgery. HIV had struck the country with a vengeance, and we were told to avoid elective surgery until the safety of the blood supply could be assured.

So we waited. In retrospect we were fortunate – many people who had surgery, elective or non-elective during this period, were exposed to the HIV virus from the blood supply. Jennifer had to continue to contend with the stoma and draining bile, but she was not exposed to a contaminated blood supply.

We waited, until she was forced to have surgery to remove her enlarged spleen. Fluid had accumulated, and her spleen had become five times the normal size. She was at risk for hemorrhaging. The window of waiting had closed, and we were thankful they felt the blood supply was no longer at risk. She would need a large number of units of blood on reserve during the surgery and would have been at a great risk for exposure to HIV. Any surgery is risky, and for Jennifer it has always been more so. They would close the exterior stoma the same time they removed the spleen. Jennifer was very familiar with the discomforts of surgery but went into this surgery enthusiastically – she would be getting rid of the stoma. If the surgery went as planned, no longer would she be faced with bile draining from the stoma.

Many people live full lives without their spleen, but there are precautions that need to be taken. The spleen, little understood until the past century, plays a vital role in the immune system's response to disease. It is also involved in the blood's ability to clot. It is a reservoir for white blood cells and platelets, and although the jobs of the spleen are taken over by other systems and organs, the loss would mean she was more susceptible to illness. Many people lose their spleen to dramatic injury such as in a bad fall or car accident, and others are removed due to illness. Jennifer's had been compromised due to the increasing size of her abdomen. Blood was backing up in the spleen, and she was in danger of hemorrhage. What were the precautions she would need to take following surgery? She would be more susceptible to infections, particularly a type of pneumonia that could quickly overwhelm her system. She would need to take the pneumococcal vaccine, every ten years, to help protect her from this particular bacteria. She would be susceptible to other bacteria and would need to alert medical personnel to the absence of her spleen. Little did we know the issue of the spleen's role in the blood clotting would be a factor down the road.

Jennifer's abdomen was a road map of surgical scars. Surgery was always more difficult due to the complexity of her illness and the scars that had to be navigated during surgery, and the map was expanding. She would be losing her spleen but gaining the independence of life without the stoma.

Laughter is one of Jennifer's trademarks. She adored watching television with her father, and there were many nights I would cook dinner and listen as she laughed uproariously at “Mama's Family” and “MASH.” **WHEN PIGS FLY** became one of her favorite expressions and she didn't hesitate to use it when someone suggested or said something she did not believe was possible or true. For all those who told Jennifer to quiet down, stop laughing in movie theaters, I would say **WHEN PIGS FLY.** Laughter got her through many ordeals and difficulties. Dr. Mendez-Picon, one of her surgeons at MCV, loved Jennifer's laughter, but when her stitches became compromised as she laughed he temporarily banned her from watching “MASH” or “Mama's Family.” She and her father were forced to watch shows that occupied her time but were not quite as funny. We made sure to tape both so she could watch them after her stitches were removed.

It was1982, and Jennifer was ten and getting ready to undergo surgery for removal of her spleen. We were delighted to add another member to our family – Jennifer's little brother Adrian. It made for a busy house, especially as Jennifer prepared to go through another surgery. Not only was she getting rid of her stoma, she was shedding the role of baby in the family. She now had a little brother to mother and love.

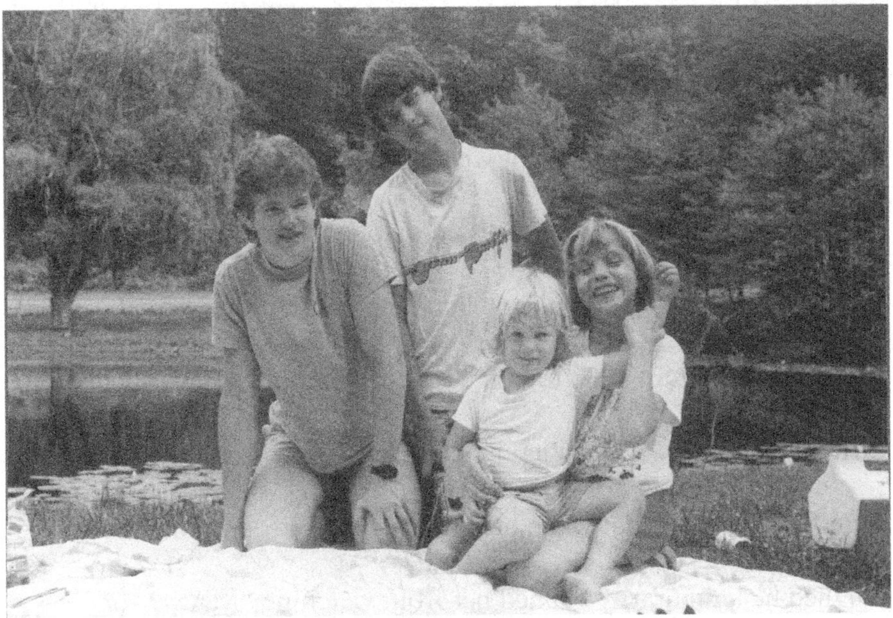

Illustration 6: Aaron, Chris, Adrian, Jennifer, 1984

Life was easier for Jennifer after the stoma was closed, but her prognosis remained the same. For the first time she was able to attend school, visit friends, and do what she wanted without the fear of bile draining through her clothing. Still jaundiced with an enlarged abdomen, she entered her pre-teen years and middle school with a little more normalcy than before.

What was middle school like? Awful. As awful as middle school seems to be for most preteens but in Jennifer's case it was even worse. We had moved to Annapolis, Maryland, in 1984, and it was here she completed middle school. Jaundiced and with the large abdomen, she was the brunt of countless comments made by contemporaries about her "pregnancy," and her "green skin." Very independent, I usually never heard of it unless the other children were particularly thoughtless and cruel.

Did she have friends? Yes, she did. She was very gregarious and would give other children the benefit of the doubt if they were unfriendly. It was often the parents who were difficult and hesitated to include her in activities. She was facing the same attitudes she had faced when she was little, but with a difference. I could not shield her from the perceptions and attitudes of people as I did when she was a younger child. She was surprisingly resilient. I am not sure I could have handled it as well, but that is Jennifer's personality – she has always been determined to not let anything stand in her way.

There were friends, some very close. The middle school years are difficult years for most children, and Jennifer and her friends were no different. There were pajama parties with preteens staying up all night talking about boys, trying new makeup, and watching movies. There was the time I came home to find myself locked out of the house. I knew Jennifer was home and could not imagine why she was not answering the door. Later I found she and some friends had been smoking and were trying desperately to dispel the smoke before I returned.

We tried to provide a normal life with normal activities, but she was still sick with a failing liver. Infections that for others would have been limited for her became quite dramatic. Something as common as a sinus infection would keep her flat on her back in bed for three or four days.

School was a challenge for Jennifer. Not because she was unable to do the work but because she was frequently sick and out of school. In addition the saying “appearances count” proved to be more than true. Some teaching personnel Jennifer encountered reacted to her appearance – the jaundice and enlarged abdomen – no differently than the children her age and some of the adults. They questioned her ability to academically perform. She was constantly forced to prove herself.

High school, for some their best remembered years. For Jennifer it would not be the case. Her liver functions had begun to decline more rapidly and she began to miss more time from school. By the beginning of her sophomore year it became more and more difficult each day to leave for school, and by the middle of the semester she was home bound.

She would have to undergo a transplant, and it would need to be done soon. Her liver was failing rapidly and would soon begin to affect other organs and systems in her body.

CHAPTER NINE

DISAPPOINTMENT AND HOPE

Pediatric liver transplantation was no longer considered an experimental procedure. The technique had been refined and most insurance companies provided coverage. Still very much a major surgery, and only performed as a last resort for end-stage liver disease, it was not the same as it was sixteen years earlier when Jennifer was born. If there was a compatible donor liver and the surgery went well Jennifer had the chance for a new life. It was a major decision on Jennifer's part as well as ours. The recipient of a transplanted organ has the opportunity for a new life, but it is also a lifetime of taking medications to prevent rejection of the organ. There is a commitment required of both the patient and their family, and some are unable to accept this. We had no problems with the concept of this commitment – we all, including Jennifer, had spent the last sixteen years committed to her well being. There was no question Jennifer would opt for the transplant – there was no alternative.

Not only are there technical and medical decisions when deciding upon a transplant, there are a myriad of psychological and emotional issues to be addressed. Although live donor liver transplants are performed today, it was not a viable option in 1990. If it had been we would have explored it, hoping either Tony or I would be suitable. We all had to come to grips with the realization that it would be the death of someone (usually from a catastrophic injury) that would enable Jennifer to have a chance at a new life. It was a sobering thought.

VCU (MCV) had an established liver transplant program and team. The physicians and surgeons on staff were familiar with Jennifer – she had been a patient there since birth. In addition we had family in Richmond. The recuperation from major surgery such as a liver transplant can be extensive, although not what we would have faced sixteen years before. We had many family members anxious to open their homes to us if we needed to stay in Richmond for an extended period of time.

Jennifer was accepted on the transplant list, and we began the wait. A wait that involved carrying a pager – remember, cell phone usage was still not that common. This was not an arbitrary decision but one of dire need. Jennifer's liver was rapidly failing. She needed a transplant before the other organs in her body began to be adversely affected by the failing liver. Jennifer was growing sicker by the day, and I never left home without it. Bags for Jennifer and for us were packed and kept in a closet, ready to make the trip to Richmond. There is a tight window of opportunity for a transplant, and the donated organ will remain viable for only a limited amount of time. In the case of a donor liver it is approximately twelve hours. A month after going onto the transplant list, the beeper sounded. Were we prepared? Physically, yes, but it was a very emotional ride to Richmond. This is what we had planned and hoped for, but it was also terribly frightening. Jennifer, if the surgery went well, would have a long road to recovery.

Once again Jennifer's seeming ability to fall outside the normal curve would play a role, and it almost cost her the opportunity for a new life. Donor livers are extensively checked before transplantation, but in a small percentage of cases they are discarded on the operating table. Upon final examination upon arrival at VCU the donor liver was not considered viable. Prepped and on the gurney waiting to go into the operating room, we were told the surgery could not be performed. The donor liver fell into the small percentage found to be unsuitable after passing the initial examination.

Dejected and depressed, Jennifer rode with us back to Annapolis, once again carrying the beeper. We were assured she would be at the top of the list, but would there be an acceptable donor in time? Jennifer's health continued to deteriorate, and we knew this was a tremendous psychological blow. Little did we know we would be faced with a major obstacle within the next few weeks.

VCU's liver transplant program was placed on hold. The liver transplant surgeon was leaving the program and there was no surgeon to immediately take over the responsibilities. They were unsure when and if the program would start accepting patients again. Where did this leave us? Scrambling to find a new group willing to accept Jennifer into their program. And it would be a group who had no immediate knowledge of Jennifer. She would have to undergo extensive testing and evaluation by a new team who had never seen her before.

We slid further from the plateau, and the slide seemed to be accelerating. Jennifer's health continued to fail rapidly, and we were desperate to get her re-listed at a transplant facility. Our comfort zone of Richmond was gone – we were swimming in unfamiliar waters. What were our options? The University of Pittsburgh was certainly an option. Dr. Starzl was renowned for his work with liver transplantation, and he had trained many of the liver transplant surgeons working in the country[v]. There was a program at Johns Hopkins Hospital in Baltimore, only thirty-miles from home. We explored that option first, knowing there would be an extended stay in the hospital and initially multiple follow-up visits.

We realized even more sharply how fortunate we'd been to have the program at VCU. They knew Jennifer intimately, and we had family in town. We would not have had to face spending an extended period of time with unfamiliar physicians and in an unfamiliar town. At least Baltimore was not as far as Pittsburgh.

We were shocked when the Johns Hopkins transplant program rejected her. Just a month before she had been ready to be wheeled into the operating room at VCU to receive a new liver, and now a team of doctors at Johns Hopkins was telling us her poor health prevented her being listed. Her poor health was a direct result of the failing liver, and she was denied the chance for a new liver and restored health. Biliary atresia is one of the most common conditions requiring transplantation, and Jennifer was a young woman, not even legally an adult. How could she not be given this opportunity at life?

It was a bitter disappointment, and without the help and intervention of our friend and family physician Dr. Victor Plavner, Jennifer would likely not be here today.

Searching the literature for available transplant centers, Dr. Plavner read of a new program at the University of Virginia Hospital (UVA) in Charlottesville, VA. It was a young team and a new program, and they quickly agreed to see Jennifer for an evaluation.

Within a few days we were on our way to Charlottesville and UVA. Jennifer had spent eight summers going to Camp Holiday Trails and knew Charlottesville well. She had made a number of trips to the hospital when she had medical issues at Camp as well as going to visit some of the other campers who had spent time at UVA. We were hopeful but also worried – what if the outcome was the same?

What a breath of fresh air. Evaluating Jennifer, Dr. William Stevenson, surgeon and a member of the UVA transplant team, reminded us Jennifer was a very sick young woman. Having said that, he told us she would immediately go onto the list . "She is 18 years old, and even if there is only 1% chance of success, she has her life ahead of her and deserves the chance for a transplant." Dr. Stevenson had trained in Pittsburgh with Dr. Starzl's program, and we were jubilant. Jennifer was going to be given the chance at life. Dr. Stevenson was young and full of energy, and we immediately felt an overwhelming sense of hope and excitement.

CHAPTER TEN

A NEW LIFE

Two weeks following Jennifer's evaluation at UVA, we received a call from Dr. Stevenson at three a.m. We had slept through the beeper. In a deep sleep, I held the phone wondering who was calling at such a late hour and why I couldn't hear them. Turning on the light I realized I was holding thc phone upside down! A donor liver was on the way to UVA and Dr. Stevenson told us we needed to get to UVA. A twelve year old girl had died and her organs had been donated for transplantation. The donor liver appeared to be a good match for Jennifer. What was our reaction? Excitement, exhaustion, and of course worry. And sorrow that a young girl had lost her life. It is a difficult concept to accept that someone's death has enabled someone else to live, and it is something we had often talked about.

Charlottesville is about three and a half hours from Annapolis, and it was morning when we arrived at UVA. We did not know where the liver came from but knew it was on its way to Charlottesville, just as we were. We were all quiet on the trip to Charlottesville. What went through our minds? Worry and concern for Jennifer.

Arriving at UVA, Jennifer was quickly taken to the operating room suite. We were left standing there, wondering if we'd made the right decisions, if we'd see Jennifer again. We'd been told due to her poor health she had a 50% chance of surviving the surgery – those were terrible odds, but it was a 100% certainty she would not live without the transplant.

Eighteen, Jennifer had to sign the paperwork for her surgery, including the consent form where she acknowledged she might not survive the surgery. How it broke my heart – we had made all those decisions in the past and signed all of the forms for prior surgeries. What a terrible burden placed upon her.

Wheeled down the hall, Jennifer called to her older brother Aaron to take care of "Fireball" - her yellow tabby cat and her talisman. As long as Fireball was with her, things would go well. He was her constant companion at home. It terrified me to hear her say that as I was afraid she felt she would not survive.

With multiple units of blood on reserve for Jennifer, the marathon surgery began. Every few hours someone from the operating theater would come to talk to us to tell us how things were going, and this continued for the next twenty-four hours. What they had thought might take twelve hours had stretched on into the next day and the next night. March 10th would become Jennifer's second birthday – her day of rebirth.

How did we spend the time? Extended family members had driven to Charlottesville from Richmond, and the number of people in the waiting area grew. Aaron, a student at VA Tech in Blacksburg, had driven from Blacksburg, getting there in time to see Jennifer before the surgery began. It was Aaron she had entrusted Fireball's care. Adrian, her eight year old brother, stayed close to the rest of the family. I am not sure we ever discussed with him beforehand the dangers Jennifer faced during the transplant – if not, we should have. Jennifer was his big sister and he adored her.

The hospital personnel were wonderful, with no comment made about the number of people coming and going. We tried resting on the benches, jumping up whenever someone from the surgical team came into the room. It was March and the weather in the mountains can be cold with snow or a beautiful Spring day. Those who smoked would take a trip to the second floor where there was a large deck overlooking the countryside for a quick smoke or a cup of coffee.

Walking into the ICU to see Jennifer after surgery, she was unrecognizable. There were tubes running in and out of her body to drain fluids and replace essential fluids. The incision was open with netting placed over it – there had been so much swelling they were not immediately able to suture the surgical would. That would not occur until the next day. There was increased danger of infection as a result, but she was receiving strong antibiotics to fight infections. We were unable to touch her except to stroke her hand. Unlike eighteen years before when she was in the sick baby nursery, all of her family, including extended family who had waited through the day and night of surgery, were able to say hello to her. I asked Jennifer later what she remembered, and she did remember everyone coming into the room to say hello – but her first reaction was to wonder where the herd of cattle had come from! Her eyes were shut and she was still under modified anesthesia, and it took a few minutes to realize we were there and talking in whispers. We never told the rest of the family Jennifer thought we were a herd of cattle!

It was here, during her stay as a transplant recipient, Jennifer made a life-long friend. Mary Douglas, one of the transplant coordinators, not only guided Jennifer and her family through the intricacies of the recovery but became a good friend. Highly skilled and trained in her field, she is also compassionate and understanding. She became a friend to the whole family, and shared Jennifer's road to recovery.

Jennifer lived up to her reputation as a fighter and was discharged from UVA in less than a month. Years before, as a baby, we'd been told she would probably spend the last six months of her life in the hospital if she underwent a transplant.

Did things go smoothly in the hospital? Yes and No. Jennifer did exceptionally well, but it is unrealistic to think someone could undergo major surgery of that nature and not face some setbacks. The transplant surgery had been extremely delicate and her intestines had been nicked. Considering the twenty-four hour marathon surgery required for her transplant it is not surprising something like this occurred. Remember, when we first saw her in ICU her organs were so swollen they had not been able to close the incision, and they had placed surgical netting over the incision site. A set-back but we felt confident her surgeon would have no problems when he went in to operate. Removing twelve inches of compromised intestines, Jennifer did well, but to this day she will tell you the pain from this surgery far exceeded the pain she experienced from the transplant itself. Abdominal surgery is known for being particularly painful, likely due to the trapped gases in the abdominal cavity.

Was this her only setback? No, and the next setback was avoidable. She had developed excessive fluid in the lungs, and one of the physicians prepared to put a tube in to drain the fluid. Mistakes occur and doctors and hospitals are not infallible, even though we like to think they are. During the procedure to insert the drainage tube into the lungs the stomach was perforated. A surgical error had been made and it was potentially life threatening. There were two options – to either let it heal on its own, which would mean an extended stay in the hospital and a slow recovery, or to do additional surgery. Jennifer made the decision to undergo the surgery. Later we were asked if we thought about suing the hospital and our response was "only if she had not survived or had long term damage from the mistake." Our goal was to have Jennifer return home healthy and ready to lead a new life, not to get involved in a legal battle with the hospital.

There are multiple medications necessary following a transplant to prevent infection and rejection. We prepared for the long-term drug regimen and agreed to work with Jennifer following surgery. The regimen, although it may vary over the years, is a life-long commitment. Although Tony and I both were part of the family team to work with Jennifer, she required very little help from us. She was eighteen, and with her spirit of determination she did a wonderful job of following the doctors' orders and recommendations.

Remarkably, Jennifer was discharged from the hospital in just over three weeks. Returning to Annapolis in April, we were greeted with the flowers and sun of spring. What was life like once we returned home? Wonderful. Jennifer started to gain weight. She had a beautiful rosy color to her cheeks – and there was no more jaundice. She was weak from the surgery but made a determined effort to build up her strength. Many transplant patients undergo physical therapy to help regain their stamina and strength. Jennifer's age was a factor in her quick recovery, but it would not have occurred without her determination to start a new life. By September she was ready to return to school for her senior year. A different person in appearance – no more extended abdomen, no more jaundice – but the same caring, determined Jennifer as before.

Senior year was magical for Jennifer in some ways and in others was a letdown. She had been through so much in her eighteen years she found it difficult to appreciate what other young women her age were concerned with. She had been to the edge and had returned, and she had different values and perceptions of what was important. It was difficult to overlook the shallowness common to young people of that age, particularly if you walked in Jennifer's shoes. Yes, looks were important. So were the school activities, many which she actively participated in. But to Jennifer they were not the most important things.

During her senior year she developed a friendship with the young man who would become her husband four years later. Going to her senior prom with Chris, she looked beautiful. This was one young woman who was not told she could not stay out all night. She and Chris welcomed in the daybreak the night following the prom. A year before she had been recovering from her March 10th transplant, and the year prior to that she had been on a list, hoping a compatible donor liver would become available in time. What were her plans after high school? She was looking forward to college and living away from home for the first time. She had to battle the misconceptions and thoughtless attitudes of many at her school, even from some of the personnel who should have known better.

Returning to school in her senior year, a teacher told her he'd not known she was so ill. How the jaundice and swollen liver escaped his attention we never knew, and he had Jennifer in two classes. It was certainly not a positive reflection of school personnel's perception of a student. One of the guidance personnel had told her when she was a Sophomore she would never go to college. She delighted in showing him her acceptance to Virginia Wesleyan College in Norfolk, VA. Once again appearances had made a difference. Here were two people in the same school setting, both seeing Jennifer on an almost daily basis, and their perceptions were entirely different. One was obviously oblivious to her health problems, the other attributing lack of ability due to her health problems. She had not been the average high school student with the typical problems of young people her age. She had again defied everyone's expectations but ours.

CHAPTER ELEVEN

MOVING ON/MOVING OUT

The beaches along the Atlantic Coast had been favorite vacation spots for our family over the years, from Virginia Beach to the Outer Banks. Jennifer knew where she wanted to go to school and it was near the water. Aaron was at VA Tech where the student enrollment was close to 30,000 students. She did not want the mountains and she did not want such a large school. She wanted a small college with more individualized attention, and she wanted to be near the ocean. Virginia Wesleyan was exactly what she was looking for. Jennifer was ready to take another step into adulthood, and one many students are afraid to take. She was going away from home and what was familiar into an entirely foreign environment. She knew no students attending Virginia Wesleyan but this did not deter her. She had been going to Camp Holiday Trails for eight years, the last as a junior counselor working with the younger campers. She was independent and self-sufficient – much more so than many young people who had never faced a fraction of what she had faced. She had traveled throughout Maryland and Virginia on trains by herself, often with a trunk or suitcases that weighed twice what she did. She had learned to make friends easily, at the same time being careful to not be influenced by material possessions. She had her health and a new life to look forward to, and that included the adventure of going away to college.

What would we have said if she'd wanted to go across country? We would have worried but how could you say no to someone who has had to make decisions as she had? We tried to let her make her own decision on where to go to school, but I was delighted she chose the Norfolk/Virginia Beach area. My twin sister was living nearby, and if any problems came up she would be there to help Jennifer. It was impossible for me to completely let go – I had spent the past eighteen years watching over and taking care of Jennifer. Adrian, Tony and I drove her to school, making it a long-weekend vacation. Meeting Jennifer's roommate, we roamed all over campus. Adrian spent the night on campus with Jennifer, staying up late to play pool with her in the campus room. It was difficult for him to go home without her. Ten years older, she had always been there for him as a big sister.

CHAPTER TWELVE

DISASTER

Jennifer was not on a plateau but at the top of the mountain. She was two years post transplant, living away from home, dating, and having a wonderful time at college with new friends. Friends who had never known her prior to her transplant and only knew her as Jennifer, another college freshman. Jennifer, standing five feet tall, became fast friends with a tall, striking, red-headed young woman nicknamed Red. She was close to six feet tall, and watching five foot tall Jennifer walking with Red was like looking at Mutt and Jeff. A year ahead of Jennifer, she was her support when anything unusual happened, and it was Red who persuaded Jennifer to get in touch with my sister when she was not feeling well.

She'd not felt well, and the physician at the College ordered lab work and other tests. Nancy, my sister, and Red made multiple trips to the hospital with her for tests, but they were unable to identify any problems and sent her back to her dormitory. Reluctantly, Jennifer knew she needed to make a trip to UVA to be seen by her transplant surgeon.

It was March, and it had been two years before on March 10th when Jennifer received her transplant. We anticipated a quick trip to see her physicians, perhaps a medication change or adjustment, and then a return to college. Unable to determine what the problem was, she was admitted to the hospital for tests and observation. Disappointed, Jennifer was hoping to return to campus by the weekend.

Within three days our world would come to a crashing stop. Jennifer did not slide off the mountain – she flew off, stepping into a dark abyss.

Sitting with Jennifer in her room early on the third day, her breathing was labored. She was not in pain but was having trouble getting her breath, and it seemed to be getting worse by the minute. Listening to her chest, the Resident on call ordered an arterial blood gas test to determine the oxygen concentration of her blood. Concerned about her condition, he ordered the results STAT and sat in the room with Jennifer until the results were available. The results were devastating. For some reason she was not getting enough oxygen and it was critical. Placing an oxygen mask over her face, they rushed her to the ICU (intensive care unit). She was furious and terrified –

she had been in ICU many times before and knew it meant she was quite ill. She could not be that ill – she was waiting to go home, to get back to college. Sitting up in bed she was crying and yelling. "I am not going to ICU, I don't need to go there." The door closed behind her, and I was prevented from going into the Unit. They did not know what was going on, and they needed to stabilize her. The Resident on duty came to the door, telling me to "Get in touch with your husband and tell him to get here as quickly as possible. Jennifer is in critical condition."

Even if I could reach Tony at work, I knew he would not be able to get there quickly. Annapolis was three and a half hours distant, and he had taken his car to be repaired that morning. Our other car was in the garage adjacent to the hospital. I had family in Richmond eighty-five miles away, but I wanted him at UVA with Jennifer and me. Unwilling to take the time to get to a car rental agency, he borrowed a car from one of our neighbors, leaving a note on their door to let them know he had their car. He and Adrian would make the trip to Charlottesville in three hours, Tony hoping if he was stopped the police would understand why he was going over the speed limit.

Jennifer's transplant surgeon, Dr. Stevenson, flew back into town that evening, two days earlier than he had planned on returning. I had only seen Jennifer briefly in ICU and was told they were doing a femoral cut-down – that had to immediately filter and re-circulate her blood. Gently rubbing her forehead, I could not believe once again Jennifer was fighting for her life and no one knew what to do. It was not until very late that evening we had some answers, and the prognosis was as awful as we could have imagined.

Jennifer had developed mononucleosis (mono), and it had not been diagnosed. Diagnosis of mononucleosis can be difficult and uncertain, and I suspect and know that at times physicians, when examining Jennifer, will look for the obscure and exotic problems. They will unintentionally overlook the more common illnesses. Even if it had been diagnosed, the physicians would not have been prepared for its effect upon Jennifer.

The use of Cyclosporine and other drugs designed to suppress the immune system is not without risks, and some of the side effects were not recognized at that time. Even if mononucleosis had been diagnosed earlier, physicians did not realize Cyclosporine needed to be temporarily discontinued with a diagnosis of mononucleosis.

Maintaining a certain level of the drug in the system is important to prevent a rejection of the transplanted organ – this was something new and unknown. Maintaining the level of the Cyclosporine had caused the mono gene to morph into an Epstein Barr gene, which then morphed into a lymphoma gene. Cancer. And the lymphoma gene had morphed into Burkitt lymphoma[vi], a terribly aggressive and fast acting cancer. Tumors were all throughout her body, and they were breaking down so fast her kidneys had not been able to filter them out. That is why they had to filer and re-cycle her blood. She was in grave danger and would spend the next three and a half months fighting for her life at UVA Hospital.

What is Burkitt lymphoma? It is an aggressive cancer that frequently affects immuno-suppressed patients. HIV patients are particularly susceptible to it. Jennifer was not an HIV patient but she was chemically immuno-suppressed to maintain the transplanted liver. The HIV patient is immuno-suppressed due to the effects of their illness. But the effects were the same – Burkitt lymphoma is horribly aggressive and fast acting.

What were her options? There was only one, and it was horrible. She would have to immediately start on a devastating course of chemotherapy designed to destroy the cancer cells. We were told she might not survive the regimen of chemotherapy, but she would not survive the next twenty-four hours if she did not undergo treatment. Once again Jennifer was in uncharted waters. At the time she was diagnosed they were just beginning to identify the effects of mononucleosis upon immuno-suppressed patients. Her physicians were able to determine there had recently been a few cases, but the success rate of recovery for these patients was very limited.

Yet again Jennifer beat seemingly insurmountable odds – she survived. What were those three and a half months like? How to describe the absolute horror of aggressive chemotherapy? Designed to kill cancer cells that are multiplying out of control, the drugs are toxic. In a private room, Jennifer would not step outside the door of her room for over three months. Too weak to walk, she remained in bed. Nauseated, she could not eat and would lose twenty-five pounds. And she was bald. Totally bald from the aggressive chemotherapy. We had been forewarned, but it was still a tremendous shock. She did not lose her hair in bits and pieces. It was as she was scalped – one day her hair just separated from her skull. I was horrified, but by that time Jennifer felt so horrible I am not sure it affected her as it did me. She lay in a darkened room – the light bothered her eyes and she could stand no noise. The smell of food sickened her. Even the smell of popcorn cooked by the nurses would turn her stomach, and they were good enough to use a microwave far distant from her room for their popcorn. She was so immuno-suppressed from the chemotherapy no plants were allowed in the room. The honeysuckle had started to bloom and we wanted to bring some to her room to give her a smell of Spring, but it was forbidden. She loved visitors but did not want people sitting around and chatting in her room. Some people handle nervousness by chatting – she could not stand the noise. She did not talk much at all, and I don't ever remember her asking “why me.” It must have crossed her mind. The only exceptions were her friends from college and her boyfriend Chris. Red and Kirby, two close friends from Virginia Wesleyan, made the trip from Virginia Beach to Charlottesville a number of times. Other friends from college also made the trip. Towards the end of her stay at UVA they would put her in a wheelchair, taking her downstairs to the Cafe for some privacy away from the hospital room. Chris, the most important of all her visitors, would drive from Annapolis. I never asked Jennifer what they talked about. She was very private about her relationships and I never tried to intrude. Her close friends provided a sense of normalcy – they were life outside of all she was going through in the hospital.

Afraid she would not be there if I left the hospital for more than an hour or two, I slept for three months on two straight backed chairs pushed side-by-side, in a corner of her room. A private room, it was small and there was no bed for a family member. How could I leave for Annapolis when they could not tell me if she would survive the night? Tony and Adrian remained in Annapolis, visiting on weekends. They learned to love tuna and cheese casserole – a staple for the many nights they cooked for themselves. It was rough on them to return home to an empty house when they left on Sundays. It was difficult for everyone.

Extended family from Richmond and Maryland visited on the weekends, and my brother Jim made a date for every Wednesday night. A lawyer, he would drive from Richmond and sit with Jennifer so I could get out and walk around Charlottesville. If she was upset or feeling particularly bad, he would wrap her in a blanket and hold her on his lap while I was out. One Wednesday night when I was out he was holding her and she became violently nauseated. The nurses told me later he was so cool and collected. They provided some scrubs for him, and he changed from his beautiful suit in Jennifer's bathroom into the loaned scrubs.

My twin would show up in the middle of the night, and we'd sit on the deck outside the second floor and visit, sometimes with a glass of wine or a can of beer brown bagged into the hospital. It was Spring and beautiful in Charlottesville – it was hard to not be bitter with Jennifer in her room fighting a battle to stay alive. Relatives tried to relieve the tedium and monotony of life in the hospital, but it was difficult for me to enjoy more than short periods away from Jennifer's room. Jennifer was too ill to be aware of all of the thoughtful things done for her, but it gave me a break, if only for a very short time. Her three cousins, visiting with my older sister Lis and her husband Dick, arrived with a picnic basket packed to the brim. We sat on the deck, enjoying the delicious picnic food, but I barely ate – it was difficult to be out in the beautiful weather when Jennifer was so ill. Her cousin's husband had recently returned from flying helicopters in the Gulf War and was not allowed to visit Jennifer. He was experiencing an unexplained rash, and she was too weakened to be exposed to anything that might be contagious.

We were fortunate to be close to Richmond and so many relatives. Everyone did what they felt comfortable doing, and it meant a great deal to Jennifer to know everyone cared. Her Uncle John made the effort to bring her eighty-five year old great aunt to visit. Jennifer was so ill she was not able to speak, but it meant a lot to her. She was the sister of Jennifer's grandfather, and she had adored him. The hospital understandably can be a very depressing place, particularly on the weekend when there is limited staff on duty and it is more of maintenance of the patient's condition. It was a morale booster for me also, to know there were so many people who cared and took the time to visit.

Jennifer beat the odds and was going home. Late in July, her father carried her into the house in Annapolis after three months in the hospital. Bald and weighing seventy-eight pounds, she was too weak to walk. She had spent all of Spring in the hospital and was coming home to the heat of summer in Annapolis. Once again she was forced to depend upon me. How difficult it was for her after the freedom of living away from home and going to college. Determined to not use the walker they had suggested, she would walk down the hall from her bedroom to the bathroom holding onto the wall. Extremely weak, she fell walking to the bathroom the first night home. I lay in bed in the room across from her, holding my breath, hoping she would not fall again. She was determined she was going to regain her strength on her own and refused any form of physical therapy. It was sometimes difficult for medical personnel to accept Jennifer's determination and independence. I had to intervene to tell them to not harass her – to give her a chance to do it on her own. They were determined she would need physical therapy, but she proved them wrong – she did it on her own.

Jennifer:

How did I survive over three months in the hospital? I had no choice. I had grown so weak I was unable to leave the bed. I lost all of my hair, including my eyelashes. I was on morphine for the pain and was in danger of becoming addicted. I couldn't bear any direct light in the room and hated to hear people talking, even in normal tones. The smell of food made me sick to my stomach, and I wouldn't let anyone eat anything in the ante-room adjacent to my hospital room. All of my senses seemed to be acutely heightened. I don't know if it was the medication but all I wanted was to be left alone.

I had visitors no one else saw, such as my grandfather who had died ten years before. Mom asked me what I was saying one day, and I told her Papa had visited. I didn't tell her until later he had told me I would be all right, and Chris and I would have a life together. Was he really there? Was he giving me strength and hope to go on? I am not religious at all – I can't accept the concept of a higher being who would allow innocent people, especially children, to be sick or injured. But I am sure I talked with Papa. Was this an apparition due to the medicine I was taking? Was Papa the Third Man John Geiger writes about in **The Third Man Factor: Surviving the Impossible**? Ernest Shackleton, polar explorer, coined the term the Third Man to identify the force, being, or entity people who have survived near death sometimes experience. I am sure Papa was my Third Man. I was on morphine for a period of time, but Papa visited me before I was on morphine. Morphine is potentially addictive, and they eventually switched me to Marinol, a synthetic derivative (synthetic THC) of Marijuana. We had never heard of Marinol but it certainly helped me when I was in such pain. Driving to Charlottesville for a check-up a month after my hospital discharge, we saw a truck flash by on the highway. What did the license plate say? MARINOL. Mom and I got into a fit of laughter. We were sure whoever approved vanity license plates had no idea Marinol is a derivative of Marijuana.

I was so sick at first only family visited. As I started to improve, my closest friends from college, Kirby and Red, came to visit, sometimes bringing other friends. But the most important visitor was Chris, my boyfriend. He was a year behind me in school, finishing up his senior year in high school. We were supposed to go to his Prom in May, but I spent the night of his prom in the hospital, fighting the effects of the chemotherapy. His parents were very restrictive in the distance they would allow him to drive. He had gotten his license about a year before, and they were not willing to let him drive the three and a half hours to Charlottesville by himself. He persuaded his mother to make the trip from Annapolis, and another time he drove with a friend. But he kept in touch, calling me two or three times every day, and sending me cards almost every day. I waited for his calls each day.

When I returned home at the end of July, Chris was over at the house the next day. From that point on we were together almost daily, either playing card games, riding to the Mall, visiting friends, or going to the movies. I was bald from the chemotherapy, still very weak, and weighed only about eighty pounds. I know my family worried about me but I felt safe with Chris. On our first trip to the Mall, when I could barely walk, Chris told Mom "Don't worry, Mrs. Cooke, if she gets too tired I'll just carry her around the Mall." I could have taken the walker they sent home with me from the hospital, but I was determined to get back to living, and I knew Chris would take care of me.

About two weeks after I got home Chris showed up with a small bundle and placed it on my lap. Chris knew how important my cat Fireball was to me. A large, orange tabby, he had always been my talisman. Moving from place to place with me, Fireball was fourteen, and Chris had decided Fireball and I both needed a gift. What should it be? What meant the most to me? Fireball. Next to Chris and my family, he was the thing that provided me the most comfort. Mostly an outside cat, he sat in the driveway and waited for the school bus every afternoon. When I was sick at home in bed he would lie on the end of my bed sleeping. Did Chris worry Fireball was getting old, and I needed to form an attachment before he was gone? I don't know, and Fireball lived for another two years, dying a natural death. Instead of a replacement, the little bundle of striped calico Chris placed on my lap became a little brother to Fireball. Steven, named loosely after my transplant surgeon, spent the next twelve years going everywhere I went, becoming the head of my feline family as the population of cats in my life grew.

CHAPTER THIRTEEN

GO WEST, YOUNG WOMAN

We seemed to always be letting Jennifer go, and it was always difficult. In September, just two months after returning home from UVA, she decided to return to school, but neither she nor we were ready for her to go out-of-town. In addition, and this was the more compelling reason, Chris had decided to stay in Annapolis and attend the community college. They were very close, and she wanted to be near Chris – but she wanted her independence.

Once again we were letting go, but at least she would be nearby. Sharing a town house with other young people going to the community college, she and Steven had their own room. The bathrooms and kitchen were shared, but she had her independence and a place of her own. Within walking distance of the college and only a short distance from where Chris lived, she was on her own again, and she loved it. It is difficult to return home after living independently, and Jennifer was no exception.

Only a few miles distant, a week went by and we did not see her. We talked on the phone every day, but she and Chris were enjoying the life of young college students. She did not have her license, but Chris was there in his VW to drive her around, Steven asleep in the backseat. When she did come home for the night, Steven would come home with her. Steven, like Fireball had been years before, was her talisman. As long as he and Chris were nearby things were good. We were delighted. Six months earlier no one would have imagined she would be alive, much less flying down the road with Chris, cat asleep in the backseat, in Chris' old VW Bug.

Why didn't she drive? The time period when teenagers are usually anxious to get their license she was fighting for her life, waiting for a liver transplant. Her priorities were different. She had looked forward to driving when she was a young teenager, but at the age of sixteen her health was in rapid decline. Material possessions were not as important to her as they were to other teenagers. I don't think you could walk in Jennifer's shoes and not have a different view on what is important. At an early age she had already lost a few of her fellow campers at Camp Holiday Trails. She had made incredible decisions most people never have to make in a life time, and had undergone medical procedures and treatments that were devastating. Life was precious. She had been to the edge and back more than once.

Jennifer: Chris and I did not live together but spent most days and evenings together at the community college, going out, and babysitting for his brother and sister. Chris had a lot of responsibility thrust upon him when his mother was deployed in the Gulf War. With a much younger brother and sister, much of the daily care fell on his shoulders. He had not had a chance to stretch his wings like I had when I went to college in Virginia, and he knew he needed to make some decisions about his future. During the Christmas break from school, he told me he was planning on going into the Air Force the following May and asked me marry him. What was my response? I was exhilarated but also afraid. I wanted to marry Chris but I was afraid of the separation required when he went into the service. We had been inseparable for nearly two years – how would I manage when he went to basic training in Texas? He was my best friend as well as the man I loved. He was the one who had been there for me every day when I needed support and love.

All these years later we laugh when we talk about January 7, 1994. Chris had taken me to Red Lobster for a birthday dinner. Little did I know what he had planned. Getting down on one knee, holding a beautiful box in one hand, he formally proposed to me again, asking if

I would spend my life with him and share his future. I can't imagine a more romantic proposal – it was something I had never let myself think about. I had dared to think of such things after my transplant but I had shuttled them back into the recesses of my mind after the cancer. After putting the ring on my finger, we tried to focus on finishing our dinner. It was difficult to do as we were excited and already making plans for the wedding we wanted to have.

Chris does not enjoy any seafood except shrimp, but I will eat almost everything from the sea. Knowing how much I love lobster, he chose Red Lobster to formally propose. Leaning closer to one another, talking, I could not believe what happened next. Trying to open my lobster I lost control of it, and a huge glob of lobster and water flew across the table, landing on Chris' face and in the middle of his shirt. Startled, Chris stood up. Mortified, I couldn't believe I made such a mess! Looking at one another, we started to laugh and could barely contain ourselves. I bet there are not many women who shower their date with lobster juice after such a romantic proposal!

Chris was planning on going into the Air Force in May 1994, and we excitedly told our family our plans. Would we get married before he went to basic training or wait until he completed basic?

Chris was anxious to finish college, and he saw his enlistment as an opportunity to acquire college credits. I would have to delay finishing until we found where he would be stationed, but we were both excited at the prospect of starting our life together. Do you know the saying a little rain may fall? Well, we didn't just have a little rain, we had a torrent.

Chris' mother and step father were opposed to Chris going into the Air Force and our plans to get married. Chris' mother was in the Navy and he bore a great deal of responsibility for watching his younger brother and sister. They were not ready for Chris to spread his wings, and it took a great amount of fortitude for Chris to stand up for what he wanted. We did not find out right away, but they were also opposed to our getting married due to my health. That was the most difficult thing to accept. We had been through so much together. We were adults and had talked through all of the issues – this was our life and our future.

Our plans for a big wedding were put on hold. It is difficult for parents to let go sometimes, and change frightens many people. This was a big change – Chris would no longer be available to help with the younger children – he and I would be living half way across country. He was spreading his wings and ready to take flight.

Chris enlisted in the Air Force, leaving for basic training at Lackland Air Force Base in Texas in May 1994. The first step – a major step towards independence for Chris. And the first step towards our life together. The separation was difficult for both of us – my father can tell you of the $400 phone bill in calls to Texas. For Chris it was truly a first – the first time he had been independent of his family and the first time since his mother had deployed to the Persian Gulf he was not responsible for watching his younger brother and sister. I flew to Lackland for his graduation, and it was my first long distance flight by myself. We both were leaving the security of our families.

Our next obstacle was the wedding. We had put it on hold but had no intention of delaying it indefinitely. Returning from basic training on September 23, 1994, my Dad and I picked Chris up at the airport. We kept our plans secret.

Sitting on the floor with Steven in my lap, I looked at the clock again. Late. Where was he? Barely sleeping all night, I had finally gotten out of bed at six. Adrian had left for school, and Mom and Dad were off to work. I don't know what we would have done if someone had decided to stay home. Showered, I rushed to get dressed and ready by eight o'clock. My dress was beautiful. Not the white dress I had planned on, but a floor length Laura Ashley dress in beautiful shades of red and black with a v-neck. Chris is almost six feet tall and I'm only five feet, but I had decided to wear black ballet type flats. I didn't know how long we would have to wait, and I hated wearing heels. It was going to be a beautiful September day in Annapolis. The tree outside my window was beginning to turn and soon would be a flaming red. An Indian summer day. A beautiful day to get married.

We had stayed up late, making sure we had everything planned and ready. We'd told everyone we were going out-of-town for the weekend and would call them that evening. I think my Mother wondered what was going on. I hated to not confide in her but we had decided this was best. Where was Chris? Another five minutes had gone by and I must have looked at the clock fifteen times in that five minutes. Almost too warm in my dress, I was afraid he'd had cold feet. Was he going to be able to carry through with it, knowing his family was opposed? It was times like this I wish I'd had a sister or a close friend to confide in. The door opened upstairs, and I heard Chris rushing down the steps.

"I had trouble getting away from the house."

Upset, I wanted to yell at him, tell him how afraid I had been he had decided against it.

Running a brush through my hair one more time, giving Steven a kiss, we were finally on our way. The morning traffic on the Severn River Bridge to Annapolis is horrible, but fifteen years ago it was not as bad. You could even find parking near the Court House, which is unheard of today.

Even running late, we were the first in line. The sun was shining on us – we had wanted to be the first to get married in Annapolis that day. I was sorry our families would not be with us, and then the excitement of getting married pushed any thought of guilt out of my mind. We had one friend as witness, but we only had eyes for one another. Grinning wildly, the ceremony was short. But that did not take away from its importance to us – to us it was a beautiful ceremony. Holding the Marriage Certificate, we knew we'd done the right thing. We would have another ceremony at a later date, and have the family there. We had done what we wanted to do and had taken a momentous step towards our life together. Leaving the Court House, we walked outside to a beautiful Fall morning. The leaves were turning, the sun was shining, and we were going to be heading South for our honeymoon. We did not stop grinning the whole morning.

What was everyone's reaction? We didn't tell anyone, not for three days. We had made plans to honeymoon in Williamsburg, Virginia, and told everyone we were just going away for the weekend. It was not until our return to Annapolis on Sunday we broke the news. My family was thrilled. I think my Mother had suspected something – it was so unlike us to go out-of-town. She never admitted as much but I always wondered if she had an idea. She was totally unprepared to find out it was at the Court House in downtown Annapolis! I know she was disappointed not to be there but we could see no other way to do it. What did Chris' family think? Initially, they were not pleased. It was very difficult to let go – perhaps it is always more difficult when the first child leaves home. It is unknown territory – one day you're responsible for someone, expecting them to follow your wishes and directions, and suddenly everything is turned upside down. Not only had Chris gone into the Air Force, he had gotten married. Did they become acclimated to the new family dynamics overnight? Yes, gradually. Visiting in Annapolis at Christmas, his family seemed to be pleased with Chris' decision to go into the Air Force and our marriage. Chris' family, along with about sixty friends and family members, celebrated our wedding at a beautiful party at the Club House in our community. I wore the same dress I had gotten married in and Chris wore his Air Force dress uniform. Maybe the wine helped, but everyone enjoyed the party and showered us with gifts and good wishes. My Mother's friend Kris surprised us with a beautiful handmade quilt for our bed. I cherish it, and realize even more as the years go by how much effort it must have taken. Hours were spent on making this special gift for us and I'm not sure she realizes how important it is to me. No one, outside of my family, had ever done something like that for me.

Chris was assigned to Scott Air Force Base in St. Louis, Illinois, for his Phase II Training, and it was an adjustment for both of us. Should I stay in Annapolis until he was settled? Should I go with him and help choose our first apartment? I would go – we had been separated most of the last four months – we wanted to be together again. I wanted to be with Chris in our first apartment. Who knew anything about Illinois? A history buff and my major in college, I knew there was a lot of history associated with it but had never met anyone from Illinois. He rented a small one-bedroom apartment, and we made plans to drive West, towing a car behind us. I had made many moves with my family and Chris had moved frequently with his family as a military brat, but this was our first move together. Being a child of a military member is entirely different from being an active member of the military yourself. We were adults and were faced with accepting responsibility for ourselves. Were we afraid? Not afraid, but we were both nervous. We were excited about having our own place and Chris was excited about his work in the Air Force, but neither of us had lived such a distance from family before. I had gone away from Annapolis to college but that had only been a three and a half hour drive. St. Louis was a twelve hour drive, and it would not be a matter of going home for a weekend. Chris had become familiar with the rules and regulations of military life, but I would be learning what it was like to be married to someone in the military. I was putting my education on hold until we were more settled and would look for a job. Chris would be busy at the Base Hospital and there would be nights and weekends when he would be on duty. I would have to learn to make new friends and occupy myself when he was on duty. In addition my health care would now be in the military and I would no longer see the doctors I had known all of my life.

The VW Bug we had spent so much time in the past two years was not going to Illinois with us and we needed a car. I didn't drive, but we needed a car to get around. My Father came through with a car, something that would get us started. An old Volvo sedan, almost as old as I was. It wasn't pretty to look at as the paint job was probably as old as the car, but he had made a lot of repairs and it would get us started. With furniture donated from both our families, we were ready for our trip to Illinois.

It was exciting and we were both happy, but it was also scary. Loading and reloading the truck, Chris and my Dad hooked the trailer with the car to the U-Haul. We were running late – everything had seemed to take twice as long as we'd planned. I had complete faith in Chris' ability to drive the truck towing the car, but I knew my Mother was worried about it. I wouldn't be able to help Chris with the driving and he had never towed a vehicle before. I was anxious to get started – it was difficult to say goodbye and I knew we'd feel better once we got on the road. The last things to load were our family members –

our cats Steven, Princess and Muffin. Steven was cool and calm – he had made many trips with me in the car around Annapolis, plus he was just this laid back cat. Nothing bothered Steven. Princess, a small female tabby, was another matter! Skittish to begin with, she was terrified when we put her in the cat box in the truck, meowing at the top of her lungs. When Chris started the motor it became even worse and we wondered if we would spend the whole trip with her crying. Normally cool and calm Steven decided Princess might know something he didn't and began to howl. Luckily the noise of the truck's motor blunted the screeching – we could only hope they would eventually calm down.

We could have waited and left early the next morning, but it would have been as hard to leave then. Almost dark, we promised everyone we would stop for the night along the way. Neither of us had cell phones – who really used them in 1994? Certainly not a young married couple with barely a penny to their name! The family would have to wait to hear from us when we used a pay phone.

We were on our way. Were we happy? Yes, and excited. It was an adventure. We were truly on our own for the first time. Exhaustion did not set in until we had been on the road for a few hours. We had gotten a late start and Chris had made a point to go slowly, getting used to driving a truck towing a car. Four hours and not many miles behind us, we decided to stop for the night, hoping we'd be more rested the next morning. Chris was expected to report for duty in two days – we were cutting the time really close.

Motels were few and far between and we despaired of finding one that would accept pets overnight. Steven, Princess, and Muffin had never slept anywhere but in the house and we weren't about to leave them in the truck overnight. Besides, they were capable of making so much noise we'd probably get a call from animal control. We finally located a hotel where we were able to sneak the cat carriers into the room without the hotel employees seeing us. Setting the alarm for six o'clock, we'd be gone before anyone would be the wiser.

Struggling to wake when the alarm rang, I patted Steven, asleep between the two of us. Purring loudly, he was his usual calm self. Muffin was asleep on the chair across the room. Sitting up, I called for Princess. I wasn't surprised she was not on the bed – she was very independent and liked to curl up by herself. Tiny, she was easy to miss until she streaked across the room if you were someone she did not know. No response. Calling Chris, we searched the room and bathroom. Gone. Had someone opened the door during the night? Had she sneaked out when Chris went to check the truck? We walked through the lobby of the motel, calling her name. Had she gotten outside? Here we were, in a motel that did not allow pets, and we were looking for our lost cat! What did the hotel management do? They actually were very nice about it – of course we neglected to tell them we had another two cats tucked away in their carriers in the U-Haul.

CHAPTER FOURTEEN

'BY GAWD WEST VIRGINIA'

We needed to get on the road – Chris had orders to report to duty in two days and we had at least ten hours of driving ahead of us. I was frantic – Princess was Steven's best friend and a part of my life in Annapolis. I couldn't drive away and leave her. Calling home in tears, I am sure my parents were terrified something bad had happened. Calm as always, my Dad tried to calm me down.

"Leave our phone number. If she turns up have them call us and we'll pick her up. She'll be fine. She's been around other cats and we all know she doesn't like dogs so she won't get too close to any unfriendly dog."

I knew we had to get on the road but it was hard to leave without Princess. I wished she was in her carrier screeching – I felt guilty about letting it bother me the day before.

My Dad told me later he really didn't think the cat would show up. He'd just tried to make me feel better so I could get on the road to Illinois. He'd told me to leave our number in Annapolis to make me feel better and to get us moving. Little did he know three weeks later he'd get a call from the hotel saying they'd found the cat and would he please pick her up! She had been hiding in the building, unknown to the employees. What she ate or what she drank no one knew, but she seemed to be in good shape. It was a three and a half hour drive to Beckley, West Virginia, for Dad and Adrian to pick her up at the hotel, and from then on she became not Princess the cat but “By Gawd West Virginia” the cat – for the state where she'd lived in a motel for three weeks! Fifteen years old, frail, and even smaller than she was as a young cat, she lead a full life and was with us until 2010. Steven, my soul mate and talisman, is gone, but we had many adventures with him before he died.

Bereft about the loss of Princess, we continued on our way to Illinois. Steven and Muffin were restless. I'm sure they wondered where their buddy had gone.

CHAPTER FIFTEEN

MILITARY LIFE

When I say Chris had rented a small, one bedroom apartment before he had returned to Annapolis, I was not exaggerating. It was small – tiny might even be the word for it. Located off- base, it was a short ride for Chris to get to work at the base hospital. I had seen pictures but had not had a chance to see it. Our furniture was hand-me-downs from both sides of the family, with over-stuffed chairs and a sofa. Definitely too much for such a little apartment, and we quickly had to make decisions about throwing stuff out.

I had never been to Illinois and had never even really thought about that part of the country. What were the people like? It was winter – were we going to be locked in with snowstorms for the next couple of months? I had grown up on the East Coast not far from Washington, D.C., and gone to college nearby. I felt like we were stepping into the unknown.

It was a long day of driving, but we did not lose any more cats! Steven stayed in his carrier, using a litter box set up behind the seat of the truck cab when we stopped to eat. Muffin was new to our family, but she traveled well and quickly learned to use the cat box on wheels! It worked well but we made sure to empty the box and put both cats back in his carrier before we took off again. Every time we got back on the road after a stop Steven would howl, eventually settling down with only an occasional meow.

What did I think of the apartment? I loved it. It was tiny, but it was ours. Tiny kitchen, small living room, tiny eat-in dining area, single bath, and small bedroom. But perfect for us. Everything was new – married life, a new city and state, and life in the military. Chris had an easier time adjusting to life in the military. He had moved around the country with his mother and step-father, both serving in the Navy. I had moved usually every three years with my family, but not as a member of the military. It was related to new job opportunities as well as graduate school for my father. It was an adjustment for me to realize my identity was almost a sub-identity of my husband, the service member. Any thing I did reflected on him and I felt like I had no control over my life. Used to choosing my own physicians and having more control over my medical care, it was an adjustment to relegate my health care to military personnel. Five feet tall, blond, and less than 100 pounds, I have always had trouble with people recognizing I was an adult and older than I looked. Independence and self-reliance were forced upon me by my health problems and isolation from a typical childhood, and it was definitely an adjustment for me as a military wife.

Once people realized I was in my twenties I was constantly quizzed as to why I did not have children. I felt people were being nosy and intrusive. Chris and I had decided to wait until at least five years before we tried to have a child, and we were not even sure I could successfully carry a baby to term. It was almost as if you were the wife of an enlisted man you were expected to start having babies right away. It angered me. I was constantly quizzed about our plans for children. I had always wanted to be married and have at least two kids, but with my health always in jeopardy when I was younger I did not know if that would ever happen. The liver transplant had no bearing on my ability to bear children, but what happened two years later did. When I developed the lymphoma two years following my transplant the idea of kids went out the window. The doctors were honest with me. I needed to wait at least five years post cancer and even then I might not be able to conceive and carry a baby. I had undergone extensive and drastic chemotherapy treatments, and there was the possibility they had rendered me sterile or had damaged my eggs. I was told to wait at least the five years and to undergo testing before I attempted to become pregnant. Chris and I had talked about it extensively and had decided to wait at least five years after our marriage – seven years after the cancer treatments. What right did complete strangers have to know my personal information? It angered me but it was a constant refrain from other young women I met when Chris was in the military. I tried to be diplomatic but I know sometimes my irritation at people's lack of sensitivity showed through.

I learned to adjust, and learned to live within the confines of military expectations. We both grew to love Illinois. I had never really thought about what Illinois and that part of the country was like, but I found I loved it. The people were friendly and welcoming, and the climate was little different than Annapolis. We both missed Annapolis and our families, but we loved getting to know the people in Illinois and loved our independence. My little brother flew by himself to visit us, and we got to show him the Arches and around our town. My Mom flew out to visit, and my Dad would end up driving a car to Illinois for us. The old Volvo had finally given out, and Chris did not have the skills my Dad did to keep an old car running. It had been in the family for years, but we couldn't keep it running. Deciding we needed something more current, Dad chose a Honda Civic, driving it from Annapolis to Illinois. We loved showing the family our home and introducing them to the wonderful people of Illinois.

Chris's next assignment was California. What was our reaction? Chris was involved with his training and job and was excited about the move – for me it was more difficult. California was not a long days drive from Annapolis – it would be a cross-country flight for me to go home or for my family to visit. I was very close to my grandmother in Richmond and worried about seeing her. Her health was failing and I wanted to spend more time with her. I was excited about the prospect of seeing California but knew it would be a difficult adjustment to live that far away. To be honest, I was dreading it. I had become acclimated to my doctors in Illinois and had grown to really love the people and the state. I worked part time and rode my bike around base. It was small and friendly – California was far away and an unknown. My family promised to visit and told us they'd help to fly us home for holidays, but I was unhappy to be leaving Illinois.

Originally Chris had planned on going ahead to California, looking for an apartment, and having me meet him after he had gotten settled. I was not happy about the move but knew this would not work. I needed to be with Chris when he found a place to rent. We had been forewarned it would likely have to be off-base. Chris knew nothing about the area and neither did I – at least together we could make a joint decision on where to live. Moving is tough on everyone, and this move was particularly difficult for me. After a leisurely drive from St. Louis back to Annapolis, I reluctantly decided I would stay in Annapolis, at least for a short time, while Chris looked for a place to live. That lasted until Chris, stopping at Scott Air Force Base on his way across country, called me and told me to meet him at Scott via airplane the next day. He had come to the same conclusion I had – we both needed to be in California to look for housing and to get settled.

We were both glad we'd made the decision. Princess had stayed in Annapolis after her adventures in West Virginia, never going to St. Louis with us. Leaving Steven and Muffin, our two furry family members with my family in Annapolis, we had a wonderful trip driving from St. Louis to California. Although Chris had a schedule he had to keep, we had time for sightseeing in parts of the country neither of us had ever been to before. I had never been west of St. Louis – I was an east coast girl. When I was very young my parents had been advised to not travel out of Virginia due to my health and the uncertainty of insurance coverage away from Virginia. Chris had lived in Washington State with his parents but had never been to Arizona or California. Our route to San Francisco was dictated somewhat by what Air Force Bases were available along the way, and we were able to stay in Base hotels every night except one.

There were disadvantages of California, many we had anticipated. The distance to visit family, the higher cost of housing and other living expenses, and the difficulty of finding off-base affordable housing for enlisted personnel were a few. Did we become acclimated and learn to enjoy our stay in California? We did, and for the most part we enjoyed our stay. The weather was beautiful, and we both loved San Francisco. We visited Alcatraz, and even slept through an earthquake! We had a beautiful apartment with a swimming pool, and with the warm sunny days we spent lots of our free time beside the pool.

Chris and I both took classes at the local community college, and I worked part time on the base. As an enlisted personnel there was never enough money – frequently barely enough to buy groceries. As a young, newly married couple we probably were no different than most newlyweds, and it seems everyone has stories to tell of their early years. I learned to have a great deal of respect for the enlisted personnel and admire their ability to get by on very little money. It was especially difficult for the ones with young children. Although I would get irritated by the comments from people quizzing me about our plans for a family, I worried about the young families with children and barely enough money to scrape by. Chris and I tried to economize – a difficult concept when there is not enough money to start with. We laugh at some of the things we did when we were first on our own. For one holiday Chris had gone shopping for groceries. We both wanted to have a ham for the holidays and to enjoy later. Returning home, Chris proudly showed me his purchase – an uncooked ham! Neither of us had bothered to ask what our Mother's usually cooked, and it wasn't until we read the directions that we realized this wasn't the same kind of ham! After talking to them we realized they had always warmed a pre-cooked ham. We celebrated the holiday meal at the Golden Arches!

Muffin and Princess, or rather 'By Gawd West Virginia,' were really outdoor cats and had settled to living in Annapolis. We were anxious to have Steven and a new black kitten named Midnight join us in California. On a visit back to Annapolis, we decided to fly them back with me to California. My Mother and I have laughed whenever we think about Steven's trip to California. Steven, Chris' gift to me, was three and had grown into a plump, no, overweight cat, and Midnight was a tiny three month old jet black kitten. Steven and Midnight would fly in the same cage on the floor in front of my seat. We never figured out what the air port screener was thinking – this was at least five years before air port security was tightened, but we were told to take both cats out of the cage before I could board the plane. The plane was getting ready to board, and I was afraid I would miss the flight. They insisted they had to run the wand under Steven's abdomen! I guess he was so plump they worried he might be carrying something! Here we are, my mother and I taking Steven and Midnight out with the screener running the wand back and forth under Steven's plump tummy. A normally cool, laid back cat, Steven decided he had been subjected to enough indignity, and letting out a screech, became stiff as a board.

"He's good to go" was all the screener said as she waved us on, but Steven would have nothing to do with returning to the cage. We'd slipped tiny little Midnight back into the cage, but Steven was spread-eagle across the cage opening, refusing to let us pry his arms and legs away from the opening. Terrified and stiff as a board, every time we'd get one leg loose he would immediately stiffen up again, and go spread eagle across the opening. They were calling for the last boarding of my flight, and all I could think about was getting on the plane and all Steven could think of was not going into the cage! By the time we got Steven into the cage the contents of my backpack were scattered over the floor, my mini skirt had hiked up, my blouse was covered in cat hairs, and my hair was plastered against my face! Did we make the plane? Yes, but only by running down the concourse. My Mom was not ticketed so could not go the last part of the concourse, and I am only five feet tall and weighed about ninety-five pounds. We have laughed often, but all I remembered thinking was "when we get to California you're on a diet Steven – enough is enough." He had to weigh at least twenty pounds, and poor little Midnight was sliding from one side of the cage to the next as I ran to catch my flight! I guess he was exhausted, as I barely heard a sound from him all the way across country, and lucky for my fellow travelers he did not need to use a cat box! I would occasionally hear a little meow from

Midnight, but Steven, reverting to his cool and calm personality, put his paw on her and licked her face until she quieted down.

We had decided to wait on trying for children, and perhaps that is why our cats were such a big part of our family. Not only did we have Steven and Midnight, we added an eight week old yellow tabby I named Furball. Steven, named after my transplant surgeon William Stevenson, was always the king of the pride, but Furball became my replacement for Fireball, my orange tabby from my childhood. I spoiled him completely, taking him everywhere as if he were a baby, and he responded with total devotion. He was a talker and seemed to always know when I needed special attention, settling beside me or on my lap. I do think animals, and some more than others, seem to be aware of people's thoughts and feelings. On my Mother's first visit to see us in California she slept on a sleeping bag in the small second bedroom. The next morning she told me how strange yet comforting it had been – Furball had spent the whole night, sitting straight up, meowing and talking to her all night. It was good she was an animal lover, as Furball barely left her side the whole time she was there! I think it was because he and my mother were tuned in to me and my feelings – they both loved me.

Our family continued to grow with the addition of two brothers – Peanut and Niko. Both male, Niko had long white fur that touched the floor. Peanut was the image of my Grandmother Mary's cat – a beautiful Maine Coon cat. We were allowed to have pets in our apartment, but I'm not sure the manager of the complex ever realized how large our family had grown!

CHAPTER SIXTEEN

RETURN EAST

We made new friends and got to know a fascinating part of the country, but we were anxious to go back East. Both our families were on the East Coast, and we decided after Chris' discharge to return home. We would miss the beautiful weather and countryside of the San Francisco area, but to us it was not home. It was winter and the weather was unpredictable, but here we were, traveling across country in our Honda Civic with our large family of cats. Steven and Midnight had flown to California, but we now had the three additional cats to manage on a 3,000 mile trip. Were they good? Yes, definitely. Steven was his usual calm and collected Buddha type of personality. Midnight was happy just to be around Steven, and Furball was happy as long as I was close by. Peanut and Niko would occasionally crawl up to Chris' shoulders and fall asleep for long periods of time. I still did not have a driver's permit, so all of the driving was left to Chris. Cat boxes were kept at the very end of the car, and were changed at least once a day. We had cat carriers for all of the cats and they would often crawl into them and fall asleep. We even made a point to detour to see the Grand Canyon. We knew we would likely not be back in the

West for a number of years and didn't want to miss the opportunity of seeing it. It was well worth the detour, and we were right – we haven't been any further West than Colorado since our return to the East Coast.

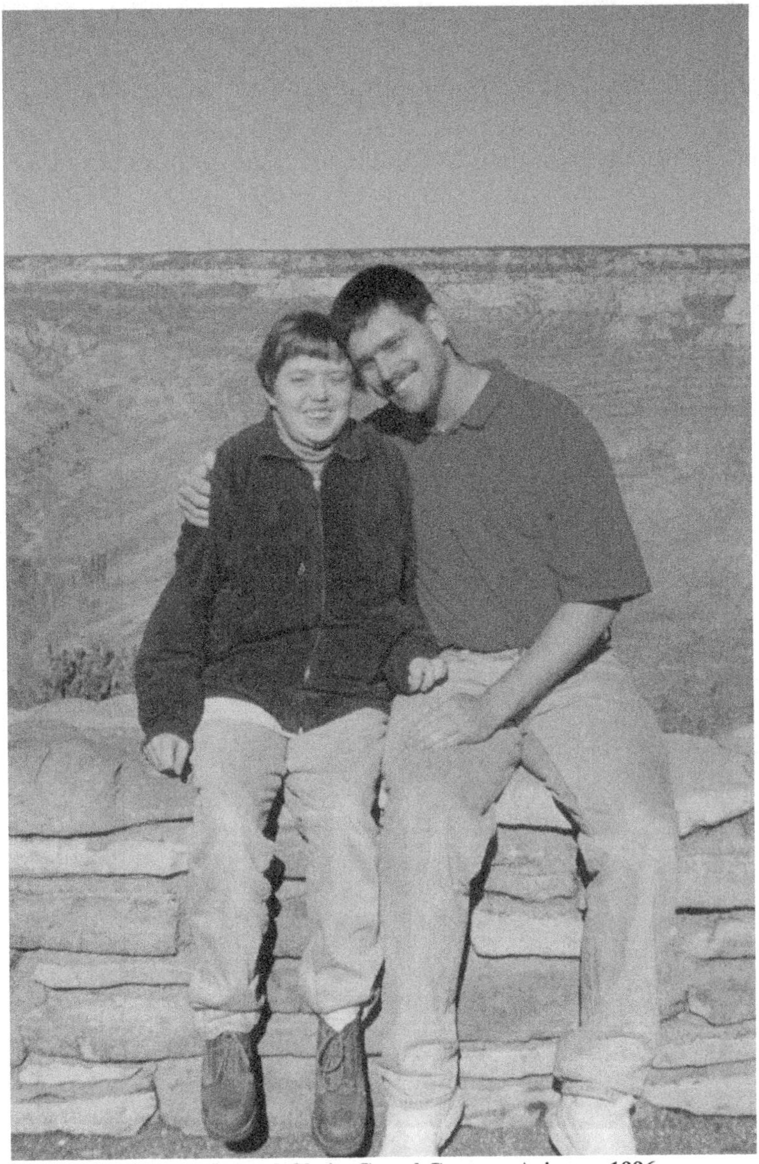

Illustration 7: Jennifer and Chris, Grand Canyon, Arizona, 1996

I wish I could say the trip was totally pleasant and uneventful, but that wouldn't be the truth. It was pleasant and we had the opportunity of seeing more of the country, including an unexpected extended stay in Albuquerque, N. Mexico. The Honda, which had never had any problems in the past two years, decided it wanted a break from the long trip across country. Fortunately it decided this in Albuquerque, but unfortunately it was on a weekend, forcing us to spend two extra nights on the road. I say fortunately as it gave us an opportunity to spend more time in Albuquerque, and we both decided we loved it. So much so we knew we might want to live there someday. We would get settled back on the East Coast, but would keep the thought of Albuquerque in the back of our minds – who knows, perhaps someday we would live there?

Change is ever constant, isn't that the saying? It had been difficult to become acclimated to life in the military and it was an adjustment to return to civilian life. It had been hard to accept the control the military exerted over everything you do, but it is a big change once it is not there. Once again I was forced to decide on physicians and health care, and a different type of control was now exerted. When I was younger, under an insurance policy that was quite good, I had a great deal of choice in my medical care. By the mid to late nineties that had changed and it was becoming increasingly dictated by the insurance companies and the type of policy you had. They dictated who you could see and where you could go. Once again I had to find physicians who understood my medical issues and recognized my ability to make my own decisions. I was fortunate we had decided to move to the Northern Virginia area, where there was an abundance of physicians to choose from. If I was displeased with a physician or a location, as long as it was acceptable with my insurance carrier, I was able to go to another physician. As long as my physicians accepted what Dr. Stevenson and I had agreed upon years earlier – "if it works, don't change it" – there was no problem. I had a few issues with physicians deciding they wanted to change my prescriptions, wanting to try me on entirely different protocols and transplant medicines. If the physician and I were unable to come to an agreement to maintain my medications as they were, I quickly looked for another more understanding physician.

Some physicians have a great deal of difficulty accepting my knowledge and ability to handle my own health care. Part of that may be due to my size – five feet tall and I have never looked my age. Part of it is the arrogance of some physicians – the god mentality. They obviously are quite bright and highly trained, but they have a very difficult time accepting my credentials as a long term transplant patient who has made a point of understanding and managing her own health.

I was lucky my parents had good insurance coverage when I was younger, and it dictated some of Chris' job choices after he was discharged from the military. I obviously had been covered for my medical care while in the military, but now we were responsible. One of the primary issues Chris looked at when he was job hunting was whether it had good insurance coverage. Transplant medications are extremely expensive, and we needed to make sure we could pay for them. My parents had maintained a private personal major medical policy on me since I was married as a fall back, but it would barely cover one month's Cyclosporine if I had to use it. Chris was able to get a job with good coverage but it still today plays a part in any decision he might make about a job change. I feel sorry and worry about people who need a transplant or have undergone a transplant and don't have good coverage. Where do they turn when they need to get their medicine? I have heard horror stories of transplant recipients cutting their daily medications in half to extend the time. What happens? They frequently go into rejection.

What were the next few years like? We did what other young couples do. We had an apartment, enjoyed vacations at the ocean and flying to Colorado to see Aaron, and moved up to a larger, nicer apartment as we became better established. I worked part time and Chris worked full time. I did work full time occasionally but my health would eventually become an issue. I suffer no ill effects from the biliary atresia, but as a transplant recipient I am more susceptible to infections. When I do get something such as a sinus infection I am usually sicker and for a longer period of time. This became an issue when trying to work full time and I found there were few employers who were sympathetic. My Mother has told me she faced the same issues when I was younger. I was sick almost constantly before my transplant and she was never able to work full time. Even part time jobs were difficult for her as I often was in the hospital out-of-town or sick at home for weeks at a time. I was a child and obviously could not stay home by myself, or stay in the hospital out-of-town by myself. Where was I able to work where they were more understanding? At McDonald's and at WalMart. I know a lot of people have a bad impression of WalMart, but they are one of the few places I was able to work and they were willing to overlook my sometimes extended absences.

Chris and I still had our family of cats and had not planned on even trying to conceive for another couple of years. Imagine our surprise and delight in June of 1998 when we found I was pregnant, and our heartbreak the following October when I miscarried. I was told to wait at least a year and to come back for testing and a workup before another pregnancy. Once again we were faced with the real possibility I would never be able to have children, and we occasionally talked about adopting. Would I even be considered as an adoptive parent as a transplant recipient? Red, my close friend from college talked to me about being a surrogate mother, but Chris and I were not ready for that step. The pregnancy had been a surprise, and we needed more time to consider all the implications. I channeled my disappointment into working and going to school part time and decided it was time for more independence. I would finally get my driver's license. Not only would it give me more independence, it would give Chris freedom from having to constantly take me places. It had never seemed really important to me before, but Chris and I were now living in an area where I needed and wanted more independence. Perhaps even more significant was the unexpected pregnancy and miscarriage – I needed the freedom to come and go the driver's license would afford me.

CHAPTER SEVENTEEN

ISABELLA MARTA

We were busy, getting established, and only occasionally thought about another pregnancy. Was I afraid of what might occur? Not consciously, although I am sure it was just beneath the surface. It was not until my younger brother Adrian told us he and his wife Jess were expecting did it really hit me. Here he was ten years younger than I was, and they were going to have a baby. All I could think about was how nice it would be if I had a baby close in age and how nice if they grew up close like I had with my cousins. I was thirty-three, and the risks of complications for me and a baby I knew would go up after the age of thirty-five.

Imagine my surprise when I realized I might be pregnant! All the signs were there – slight nausea, cessation of menstruation, breast tenderness, but the first two at-home pregnancy tests were negative. The third was the winner – a definite positive. Chris and I were in a state of shock! It had been eight years since I had the miscarriage and we had grown complacent, not even talking anymore about having children. We both assumed it wouldn't happen, I wouldn't get pregnant again. We were excited, and very nervous. Nervous about the dangers to me and to the baby, and nervous about telling my family. They would be excited but they would be worried about my health and the health of the unborn child. How would they react? I knew they would be supportive, but they were my parents and had been there with me when I was so sick. They were bound to be very concerned.

A blood test at my doctor's office confirmed the pregnancy, but we still did not tell anyone for a few weeks as we didn't want to take away from the excitement about Adrian and Jess's baby. Let everyone enjoy their news before we told them ours. But I was excited – it had not been planned but our baby would only be four months younger than theirs. They would have the opportunity to become close – almost like twins since they would be almost the same age. It wasn't until the heart beat was confirmed by an ultrasound did we feel confident about telling our family. It was music to our ears and we were ecstatic. March has always been a special month to me – March 10th is the anniversary of my liver transplant. Here we were, the first week of March sixteen years later, listening to our baby's heartbeat! Driving from Virginia to Annapolis to tell my parents, I experienced one of the few bouts of severe nausea I was to face over the next couple of months – Chris quickly learned to stay in the right hand lane so he could quickly pull to the side of the road when I turned a certain shade of green!

What was the reaction of my family and friends? They were delighted. Concerned, but excited for Chris and me. My Mother especially worried – she had seen me go through so much and knew how upset I had been when I miscarried eight years before. Surprisingly, I had an easy pregnancy. I've heard of a lot of women, with no long term health problems, who faced a more difficult pregnancy. My obstetrician transferred my care to a high-risk group of obstetricians at Fairfax Hospital and I became familiar with the team of doctors at Fairfax. It was not as convenient from where we lived, but I knew I needed to be followed by a team with experience in high-risk pregnancies. I had always been told the liver transplant itself did not preclude a successful pregnancy, but I knew there were concerns about the medicines I needed to take to maintain the transplanted organ. Pregnancy is stressful in a normal pregnancy – would it be more stressful on me? I don't think my pregnancy was much different than my sister-in-law's except for the frequency of visits and the number of ultrasounds. I had been working full time and taking classes towards my degree, and I realized I needed to cut back. I was always exhausted and my focus needed to be on this unexpected but wonderful life growing inside! My doctors recommended I stop work, at least for the last few months, and I agreed. I knew deep inside this might be my only pregnancy, and I wanted to assure the health of the baby.

Did Chris and I prefer a boy or a girl? No, absolutely not. We just wanted a healthy baby. But I was excited when we found out it was going to be a girl. My wish was coming true – Adrian's wife Jess was expecting a little girl also. The two little girls would have the chance to become close – even closer than I had been with my cousins when I was little. They would only be four months apart! I had another secret wish – I hoped my little girl had red hair. I had always dreamed of having a baby with red hair like Aaron! She had hair – that was clear from the ultrasound, but would it be red? I am blond and Chris is brunette. The main thing, even when we talked about "what color hair, what will her eye color be, who will she look like?" was her health. And all the prenatal testing and ultrasounds were coming back with good reports. Although the doctors remind you the tests are not conclusive – there are errors and not all problems are detected by the available testing – everything looked good. After cutting back on my work schedule I felt better. I could now focus entirely on this new life. I tried to eat only what was good for the baby, and tried to put on some weight. Perhaps because I was so focused on only eating what was good – fruits, vegetables, lean meats – I never gained more than ten pounds throughout the pregnancy. I was the envy of other friends who had fought excessive weight gain throughout their pregnancy.

My family and friends, excited yet concerned, called me after each doctor's visit to see how things were going. They were going fine, although there was one thing Chris and I did not share with anyone, even my physicians. I was worried about the effects of some of my daily medications on the developing fetus, and I had without their knowledge decided to stop some of them. This is not something I recommend to anyone – it was a personal decision on my part. My liver was well established – I was sixteen years post transplant. The risk of rejection was a lot less than it would have been in the years immediately following the transplant, but I knew there was a slight risk of upsetting the applecart. Immediately following the transplant it is necessary to take high doses of the drugs needed to prevent rejection. As the years had passed the doses had been reduced for most of the medicines - most of them were serving as maintenance. Some of the prescriptions were of more concern to me, and it was those I decided to do without. I wanted to give this baby the best possible chance to come into the world a healthy baby, and although I felt the risk of rejection was slight, I was willing to take that risk. Why did I not tell my family or physicians? I knew they would be horrified and worried. The whole focus for the past sixteen years had been maintaining the transplanted organ, and here I was voluntarily doing something that might put it in danger. In every other regard I followed the doctor's orders and recommendations. Told to not travel more than an hour from home, this limited my travel to see my grandmother in Richmond or my mother in Annapolis – both within the hour's drive. Chris and I had hoped to get to the beach before Adrian and Jess' baby arrived, but three and a half hours was too far. Kendal, their little girl, was born in July, but I would not see her until she was three months old. They lived six hours away in North Carolina, and I cried when she was born and I was unable to see and hold her.

Chris and I had just celebrated our twelfth wedding anniversary when we learned of the death of his grandmother. Six hours away, Chris would have to make the trip to her funeral by himself. I was a month away from delivery, and the doctors were emphatic about my not traveling. I spent the weekend resting and reading, anxious for Chris to return. He was due back late Sunday evening, and the weekend seemed to drag on forever. He was late, and I finally went to bed, knowing he would wake me when he came in. I felt fine, but my back had been bothering me all evening, and I felt like my stomach was tight. I had so much scar tissue across my abdomen from my multiple surgeries I had trouble feeling the baby kick. More often people looking at my extended belly would see her kick before I realized she was kicking! I woke with a start when he came in, wondering why I was so chilled. It was then I realized my water had broken while I slept – my clothes were soaked. Did we panic? No, as I had no contractions – or none I was aware of. I realize now the tightness across the belly was probably an indication – that and the low back ache.

My due date was November second, and it was only October second. I didn't really think about labor as I felt no pain – wasn't labor supposed to be very painful? It was early morning, before daylight, and Chris was on the phone with the physician. No contractions and it was my first – we could wait and come into the office when they opened at 8:30. We were getting nervous, and we drove to the doctor's office, getting there half an hour before they opened. What would they do? Would they put me to bed to take me closer to my due date? One of my family members had spent the last three months of her pregnancy flat on her back in bed, and I knew how hard that was.

I still did not have any signs of contractions, and we were surprised when the doctor told us to go to the hospital. He wanted me there so they could better monitor what was going on. A month early – she would be premature. And how big was she? They can't tell reliably from ultrasound – they can estimate but sometimes they are way off. I was admitted, and the monitor they placed on my belly showed I was contracting – they had not become strong enough for me to feel! Chris quickly went outside to call his family and mine to let them know she had decided not to wait until November – we were going to have an October little girl! I was nervous – no, terrified. I would finally get to see my little girl, but I was scared. Would she be all right? We had decided on a C-section, and I had been through numerous surgeries in the past. I knew how painful surgery can be and the complications that can occur.

I am small, and always look younger than my age. People in authority have a tendency to look over me, to talk above me, thinking I am not mature. The nurses were wonderful, but I did get the sense they thought I was a lot less mature and younger than I was. Chris and I were both nervous. Chris had worked in the medical field and wanted to make sure they were doing what needed to be done for me and the baby. He had many questions for the doctors and nurses, and they at times were not very understanding of his concerns. We were shocked when one of the nurses, obviously quite nervous, told us they had never delivered a baby when the mother was a liver transplant recipient. We had just assumed they had – they were a high risk group of physicians and Fairfax Hospital is a large hospital. I imagine they had handled numerous kidney transplant patients, but at least according to the one nurse, I was the first liver recipient.

Doctors and nurses still have trouble listening to patients today. I know it was a major problem when I was little, but the problem still exists. I don't think I am the only one who is “talked over” or not listened to, but it is probably worse since I am small and look younger than my age. I ran into this again before the C-section when I was asked if I was allergic to any drugs. I am allergic to a number, such as penicillin, which was not questioned. But they repeatedly questioned me when I told them I was allergic to Lidocaine and Novocaine. An allergy to those two drugs is less common, but I suffered extreme allergic reactions to both drugs when undergoing dental treatments. Years before, after being given Lidocaine for a dental procedure, I walked out to the waiting room. By the time I got to the waiting room, I was covered head to toe in huge hives and madly itching – and I mean head to toe. Hives had sprung up under my hair and I felt like I was on fire. Fortunately the dental office was adjacent to our doctor's office, and I was immediately given benadryl and a shot to counteract the effects of the Lidocaine. Carbocaine, less frequently used, works just fine. In addition I am allergic to alum, the powder used in latex gloves to keep them from sticking. This is more commonly recognized today, but Mom told me she had a really difficult time when I was younger as a lot of medical and dental personnel did not recognize or accept such an allergy. For me it was a life threatening allergy and almost killed me. When I was about five we had gone to a family fun day in Richmond, and Aaron and I had come back with large balloons. Riding home in the car, I pretended to blow the balloon up. We were on the highway, and Aaron called to my Mom from the backseat, "Mom, Jen looks funny, her face is green." Turning around, Mom realized there was something horribly wrong. My lips were terribly swollen – so swollen the top lip was covering the nostrils, and my face was turning a shade of blue/green. Fortunately we were near an exit that took us to the Emergency Room of a hospital and I was quickly given a shot of epinephrine. Unsure of what caused such a severe allergic reaction, it was not until a trip to the dentist later did they realize I was allergic to alum. The gloves used by the dentist had the same powder as the balloon and had caused an immediate swelling of my face. Remember, there was no Internet when I was younger, and any medical research necessitated a trip to a large public or university library. Mom spent hours at libraries and said she had many "discussions" with medical personnel when they argued with her they had never heard of such an allergy.

By the time my family and Chris' family arrived at the hospital, I was scheduled for the C-section at noon. I was nervous and frightened, and Chris kept leaving the room to talk to the doctors and nurses. My Mom sat in the room with me when he was out, but I wanted Chris in the room with me. I needed Chris to be there with me. I wanted my mother and father there, but I needed Chris. We were going to have our baby, a month early, and I was worried about her. Shortly after everyone had arrived, my doctor walked into the room, obviously very concerned. Pre-op blood work indicated my clotting factor had bottomed out – I was in grave danger of hemorrhaging during the delivery. It was a life-threatening situation, and not only was I in danger – we were in danger of losing our baby as well. I had been upset and frightened before, and now I was terrified. Would Chris be left alone, losing me and the baby, or raising a daughter without me? The tension in my room was incredible, with the number of medical personnel doubling. One of the nurses rudely told my Mother she had to leave the room, later half-apologizing and telling her they had not delivered a liver transplant recipient before. This was news to us, and we never knew whether that was correct.

I was in labor and there was no choice – the baby had to be delivered. I was quickly given two units of platelets and we were told I would receive more during the surgery and following the surgery. Chris was anxious and worried and facing the very real possibility he would lose me and his little girl. My parents were not allowed back into the room when I was receiving the platelets, and Chris had been told it would be later in the afternoon when they delivered the baby – they were going to try to give me as many units of platelets as possible. Unable to be with me, my Mom and Dad were walking to the car in the parking garage to store some of the items they had brought with them when Chris came running after them, telling them they were taking me back to the OR right away – they were going to deliver the baby NOW. Rushing back to the floor, Chris was told he would be unable to be in the OR with me since they were going to have to put me under. I was frantic and Chris was angry – I wanted him with me and he wanted to be there with me. I don't know why they made that decision, but I still think he should have been allowed in the OR.

"I love you" is all I managed to say as I was wheeled into the operating room. How many times had I been in an OR, and each time felt like I was being strapped down like a piece of meat. Tears rolling down my face, I didn't know if I would live to see my baby or family, and I secretly begged Poppa and Mary to look over and take care of me and their great-granddaughter. Poppa had been with me in spirit when I had cancer, telling me Chris and I would have a long and wonderful future together. Mary was my Father's mother, and everyone always said I was a real combination of my two grandmothers – Mary and Martha. Mary had died before Chris and I were married, and I knew she would have loved her little granddaughter.

Isabella Marta was born at 5:45 p.m. on Monday, October 2, 2006. She may have been five weeks early, but you never would have guessed it. Immediately letting out a lusty cry, she let everyone know she was here, she was healthy, and she had a mind of her own. Chris was not in the room with me but at the door to the OR, and the nurse held little Isabella up for him to see. Waking up in recovery with the surgical tech repositioning my uterus, I immediately saw Chris holding our tiny, beautiful little girl. Four pounds-fourteen-ounces and twenty inches long, she was gorgeous.

"Jen, she has red hair. You've got your *red-haired* little girl!"

Chris held her close so I could give her a kiss, and she opened a pair of big, beautiful blue eyes and seemed to be looking right at me.

"I love you, my sweet Isabella!" My first kiss as a mother for my beautiful little girl!

I had an uneventful recovery from the C-Section, but Isabella ended up in the NICU at the hospital. It was not surprising, really, as she was five weeks early and a preemie, but it was difficult for Chris and for me. Her lungs were perfect – she had let everyone know right at birth, but she did have problems with a poor sucking reflex, regulation of her body temperature, and jaundice. The NICU was where she needed to be to receive specialized care, but it limited the amount of time I could spend with my beautiful little girl. I had just undergone surgery, and it was not until the next day I was allowed to go by wheelchair to visit her. The nurses were wonderful and did everything possible to let us know exactly what was going on, what to expect, and in providing emotional support. I did have one typical, and now funny, incident, where once again people thought I was younger and perhaps therefore less capable that I am. Even though I had on my identifying bracelet that showed I was Isabella's mother, one of the medical personnel in the NICU had a difficult time accepting I was really Isabella's mother. At the time I was irritated – I wanted to be with my daughter and I couldn't believe anyone would try and stop me!

No one in either of our families had delivered a premature baby, and Chris and I were in uncharted territory. The wonderful nurses in the NICU made sure we knew how to handle the additional care required for a preemie, including the extra time it took to feed her until her sucking reflex improved.

Discharged after a week in the hospital, I learned what my Mother had learned when I was a baby – it is terrible to go home without your baby. Fortunately Isabella only had to stay four days longer, but they were the longest days of my life. I was recovering from the C-Section and could not go to the hospital unless Chris drove me. He arranged his schedule so we could spend as much time with Isabella as possible, and unlike when I was born, extended family were welcome and encouraged to visit. My Mother got to finally hold this beautiful but tiny little red-headed girl – her second granddaughter in four months!

What was the first year like, and where are we now? The first year was hard – harder than it probably is on most young mothers. We laugh now, but our first road trip with Isabella was quite interesting and very scary. She had been diagnosed with acid reflex when she was in NICU, and been placed on a special formula. But it seemed to be getting worse instead of better. Visiting with Adrian, Jess, and their four month old daughter Kendal, Isabella threw up – and it was like something from a horror film. She didn't just throw up. She regurgitated her formula across the length of the room – every bit of it. We all just stared in horror – how was our beautiful little girl able to lose what must have been at least two feedings at one time? Trying a number of formulas, she was eventually able to tolerate a soy based formula. Here was Isabella, forced to use an alternative formula, just as I had to do when I was younger. Thank goodness there were more choices, and thank goodness she was not faced with a devastating problem such as I had faced. Diagnosed with acid reflux, we were told she would likely outgrow it by her first birthday.

We were told she had to remain at least at a 45 degree angle for an hour after eating so she would not throw her food up. This was difficult – she was a slow eater at the beginning and we had to constantly coax her to eat. By the time she had eaten it seemed like it was almost time for the next feeding. What did we do? All I can say is thank goodness for baby swings! She would spend the first year of her life not sleeping in the beautiful play 'n pack beside my bed but in her swing. She did not sleep in a regular baby bed until she was almost a year old.

CHAPTER EIGHTEEN

THE INCREDIBLE GIFT

Where are we now? This tiny, gorgeous little baby is now a tall, happy, active four year old. She is a picky eater but will eat heartily when she is hungry and is even starting to try new foods. She goes to preschool two or three times a week, is learning to swim, and is a normal little girl. She has many friends and does what every four year old does. She is our gift, and she would not be here except for the gift twenty years ago from a family in the midst of the terrible grief of losing their twelve year old child. The gift of a donated liver was the gift of life for me. Without the donated liver I would not have survived past my eighteenth birthday. I would not have had the opportunity to marry Chris, and we would not have shared the gift of beautiful little Isabella.

The decision to donate viable organs is a difficult decision to make, but it is truly a gift of life to those in need. I was fortunate to have a supportive family and a family financially able to provide good insurance coverage. Many are less fortunate. There are many issues regarding organ donation. With a limited number of organs available, how do you determine who gets the chance of a renewed life? Who is qualified to make these decisions regarding allocation? Organ transplantation is an expensive procedure and requires a lifetime commitment to continue with the medications necessary to maintain the transplant. When I was a newborn, liver transplantation was considered experimental. It is now a time-tested medical procedure shown to be successful. It is inconceivable to me anyone could be denied the opportunity I was given at the age of eighteen. Isabella is testimony to the value of organ donation and transplantation.

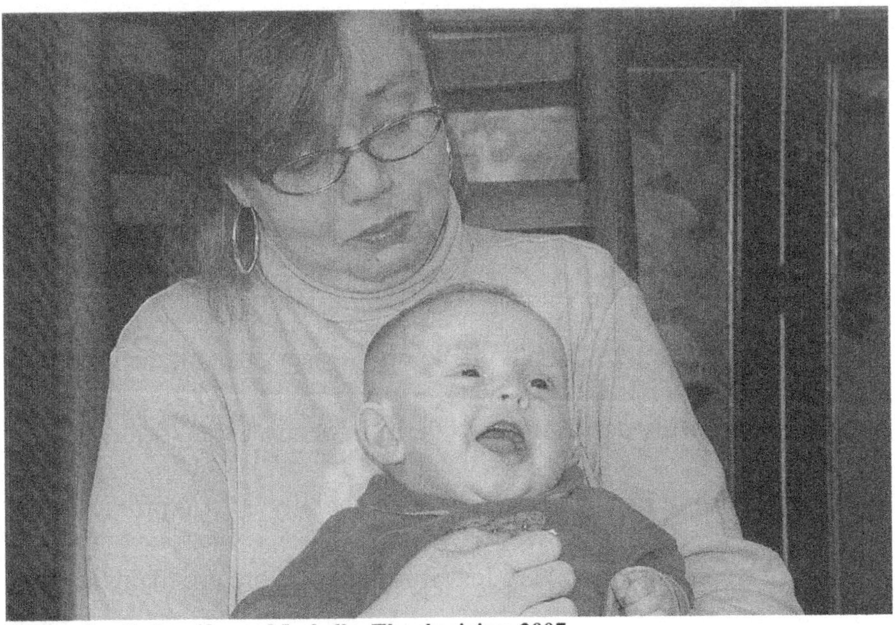

Illustration 8: Jennifer and Isabella, Thanksgiving, 2007

NOTES

For the benefit of those who are interested in more detailed information on some of the locations and medical information in **WHEN PIGS FLY** we have listed a number of resources. These are not inclusive, and a search of the Internet and libraries will provide additional information.

BOOKS

Geiger, John. The Third Man Factor: Surviving The Impossible . Weinstein Books, New York, NY 2009.

Murray, Joseph E. Surgery of the Soul: Reflections on a Curious Career. Science History Publications. Watson Publications Int., Sagamore, MA 2001

Richmond: The Story Of A City by Virginius Dabney. (University of Virginia Press; Rev Exp Su edition (September 1, 1998) (paperback).

INTERNET

Biliary Atresia:
http://www.cincinnatichildrens.org/svc/alpha/l/liver/diseases/biliary.htm
(Cincinnati Children's Hospital)

Burkitt Lymphoma:
http://www.nlm.nih.gov/medlineplus/ency/article/001308.htm

Camp Holiday Trails: http://www.campholidaytrails.org/

VCU/MCV: http://www.vcuhealth.org/
(Virginia Commonwealth University/Medical College of Virginia)

Dr. Thomas E. Starzl:
http://www.kidney.org/recips/athletics/50yrs/50yrs_pioneerBio_ts.cfm

UVA:
https://www.healthsystem.virginia.edu/internet/transplant/liver/liver.cfm
(University of Virginia)

END NOTES

i"Transplant Pioneers Recall Medical Milestones." National Public Radio (NPR). Morning edition. 20 Dec. 2004. Web. 8 Aug 2010.

ii"Liver Diseases and Treatment. Biliary Atresia. Cincinnati Childrens. Web. 9 Aug 2010.

iii_"In the Tradition of MCV. A History of the School of Medicine." Virginia Commonwealth University. Web. 5 Aug 2010.

ivLiver Diseases and Treatment. Biliary Atresia. Cincinnati Childrens. Web. 9 Aug 2010.

v"Thomas E. Starzl. Experts Page – UPMC", Pittsburgh, PA. University of Pittsburgh. Web. 5 Aug 2010.

vi"Burkitt/Burkitt Like Lymphoma,," Lymphomation Org. 4 April 2010. Web. 7 Aug 2010.

Made in the USA
Monee, IL
14 May 2026

50140908R00105